Erwin Dee Kord (Ed.)

Pericardial Friction Rub

Erwin Dee Kord (Ed.)

Solv

Pericardial Friction Rub

Heart, Pericarditis, Differential Diagnosis

Solv

Imprint

Permission is granted to copy, distribute and/or modify this document under the terms of the GNU Free Documentation License, Version 1.2 or any later version published by the Free Software Foundation; with no Invariant Sections, with the Front-Cover Texts, and with the Back- Cover Texts. A copy of the license is included in the section entitled "GNU Free Documentation License".

All parts of this book are extracted from Wikipedia, the free encyclopedia (www.wikipedia.org).

You can get detailed informations about the authors of this collection of articles at the end of this book. The editors (Ed.) of this book are no authors. They have not modified or extended the original texts.

Pictures published in this book can be under different licences than the GNU Free Documentation License. You can get detailed informations about the authors and licences of pictures at the end of this book.

The content of this book was generated collaboratively by volunteers. Please be advised that nothing found here has necessarily been reviewed by people with the expertise required to provide you with complete, accurate or reliable information. Some information in this book maybe misleading or wrong. The Publisher does not guarantee the validity of the information found here. If you need specific advice (f.e. in fields of medical, legal, financial, or risk management questions) please contact a professional who is licensed or knowledgeable in that area.

Any brand names and product names mentioned in this book are subject to trademark, brand or patent protection and are trademarks or registered trademarks of their respective holders. The use of brand names, product names, common names, trade names, product descriptions etc. even without a particular marking in this works is in no way to be construed to mean that such names may be regarded as unrestricted in respect of trademark and brand protection legislation and could thus be used by anyone.

Cover image: www.ingimage.com
Concerning the licence of the cover image please contact ingimage.

Publisher:
Solv is a trademark of
International Book Market Service Ltd., 17 Rue Meldrum, Beau Bassin, 1713-01 Mauritius
Email: info@bookmarketservice.com
Website: www.bookmarketservice.com

Published in 2011

Printed in: U.S.A., U.K., Germany. This book was not produced in Mauritius.

ISBN: 978-613-8-85830-0

Contents

Pericardial_friction_rub

A **pericardial friction rub**, also **pericardial rub**, is an audible medical sign used in the diagnosis of pericarditis.[1] Upon auscultation, this sign is an extra heart sound of to-and-fro character, typically with three components, two systolic and one diastolic. It resembles the sound of squeaky leather and often is described as grating, scratching, or rasping. The sound seems very close to the ear and may seem louder than or may even mask the other heart sounds. The sound usually is best heard between the apex and sternum but may be widespread.

Cause

The pericardium is a double-walled sac around the heart. The inner and outer (parietal and visceral) layers are normally lubricated by a small amount of pericardial fluid, but the inflammation of pericardium causes the walls to rub against each other with audible friction.

Differential diagnosis

Pericardial friction rub is one of several, similar sounds. A differential diagnosis may be possible, or not, depending upon the number of components that are audible. Pericardial friction rub may have one, two, or three audible components, whereas the similar pleural friction rub ordinarily has two audible components. One- and two-component rubs are ambiguous. A three-component rub distinguishes a pericardial rub and indicates the presence of pericarditis.

References

[1] Tingle LE, Molina D, Calvert CW (November 2007). "Acute pericarditis". *Am Fam Physician* **76** (10): 1509–14. PMID 18052017.

See also

* precordial exam

Heart

The **heart** is a myogenic muscular organ found in all animals with a circulatory system (including all vertebrates), that is responsible for pumping blood throughout the blood vessels by repeated, rhythmic contractions. The term *cardiac* (as in cardiology) means "related to the heart" and comes from the Greek καρδιά, *kardia*, for "heart".

The vertebrate heart is composed of cardiac muscle, which is an involuntary striated muscle tissue found only in this organ, and connective tissue. The average human heart, beating at 72 beats per minute, will beat approximately 2.5 billion times during an average 66 year lifespan. It weighs approximately 250 to 300 grams (9 to 11 oz) in females and 300 to 350 grams (11 to 12 oz) in males.[1]

In invertebrates that possess a circulatory system, the heart is typically a tube or small sac and pumps fluid that contains water and nutrients such as proteins, fats, and sugars. In insects, the "heart" is often called the **dorsal tube** and insect "blood" is almost always not oxygenated since they usually respire (breathe) directly from their body surfaces (internal and external) to air. However, the hearts of some other arthropods (including spiders and crustaceans such as crabs and shrimp) and some other animals pump hemolymph, which contains the copper-based protein hemocyanin as an oxygen transporter similar to the iron-based hemoglobin in red blood cells found in vertebrates.

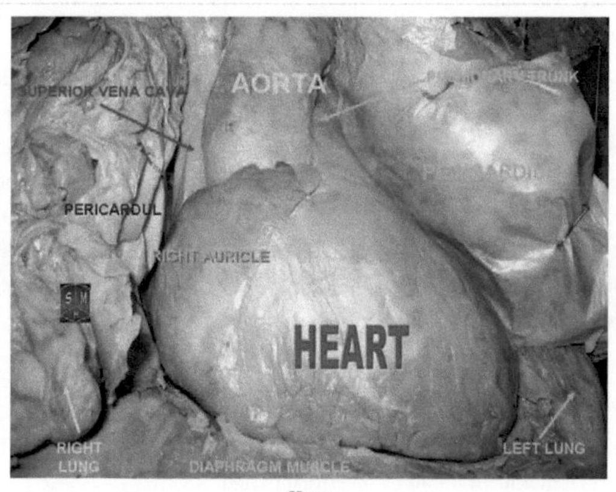

Heart

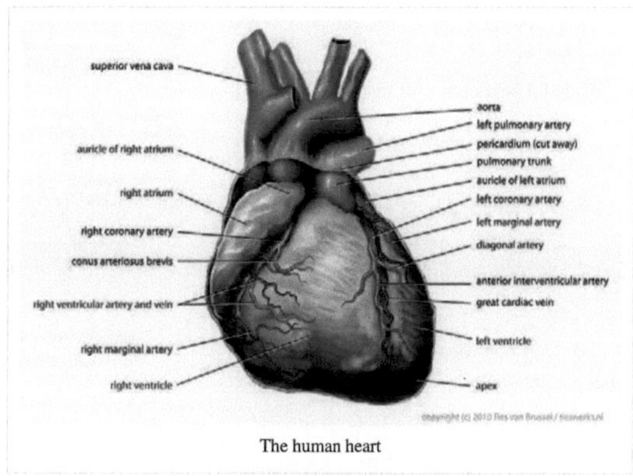

The human heart

Early development

The mammalian heart is derived from embryonic mesoderm germ-layer cells that differentiate after gastrulation into mesothelium, endothelium, and myocardium. Mesothelial pericardium forms the outer lining of the heart. The inner lining of the heart, lymphatic and blood vessels, develop from endothelium. Heart muscle is termed myocardium.[2]

From splanchnopleuric mesoderm tissue, the cardiogenic plates develops cranially and laterally to the neural plate. In the cardiogenic plates, two separate angiogenic cell clusters form on either side of the embryo. The cell clusters coalesce to form an endocardial tube continuous with a dorsal aorta and a vitteloumbilical vein. As embryonic tissue continues to fold, the two endocardial tubes are pushed into the thoracic cavity, begin to fuse together, and complete the fusing process at approximately 21 days.[3]

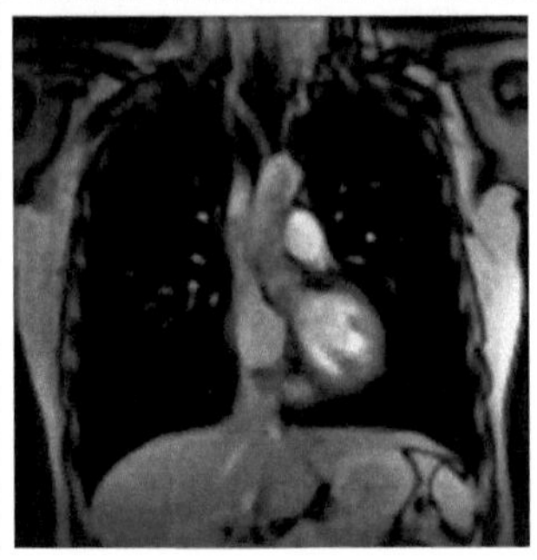

Real-time MRI of the human heart

The human embryonic heart begins beating at around 21 days after conception, or five weeks after the last normal menstrual period (LMP). The first day of the LMP is normally used to date the start of the gestation (pregnancy). The human heart begins beating at a rate near the mother's, about 75–80 beats per minute (BPM).

The embryonic heart rate (EHR) then accelerates by approximately 100 BPM during the first month to peak at 165–185 BPM during the early 7th week afer conception, (early 9th week after the LMP). This acceleration is approximately 3.3 BPM per day, or about 10 BPM every three days, which is an increase of 100 BPM in the first month.[4] [5] [6]

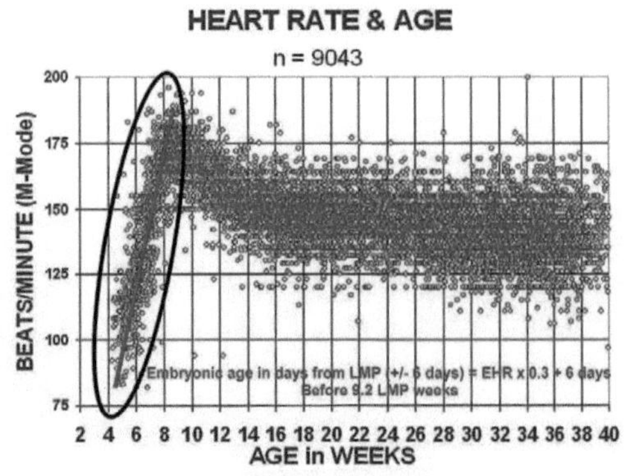

At 21 days after conception, the human heart begins beating at 70 to 80 beats per minute and accelerates linearly for the first month of beating.

After 9.1 weeks after the LMP, it decelerates to about 152 BPM (+/-25 BPM) during the 15th week post LMP. After the 15th week, the deceleration slows to an average rate of about 145 (+/-25 BPM) BPM, at term. The regression formula, which describes this acceleration before the embryo reaches 25 mm in crown-rump length, or 9.2 LMP weeks, is: the Age in days = EHR(0.3)+6. There is no difference in female and male heart rates before birth.[7]

Structure

The structure of the heart varies among the different branches of the animal kingdom. (See Circulatory system.) Cephalopods have two "gill hearts" and one "systemic heart". In vertebrates, the heart lies in the anterior part of the body cavity, dorsal to the gut. It is always surrounded by a pericardium, which is usually a distinct structure, but may be continuous with the peritoneum in jawless and cartilaginous fish. Hagfishes, uniquely among vertebrates, also possess a second heart-like structure in the tail.[8]

In humans

The human heart has a mass of between 250 and 350 grams and is about the size of a fist.[9] It is located anterior to the vertebral column and posterior to the sternum.

It is enclosed in a double-walled sac called the pericardium. The superficial part of this sac is called the fibrous pericardium. This sac protects the heart, anchors its surrounding structures, and prevents overfilling of the heart with blood.

The outer wall of the human heart is composed of three layers. The outer layer is called the epicardium, or visceral pericardium since it is also the inner wall of the pericardium. The middle layer is called the myocardium

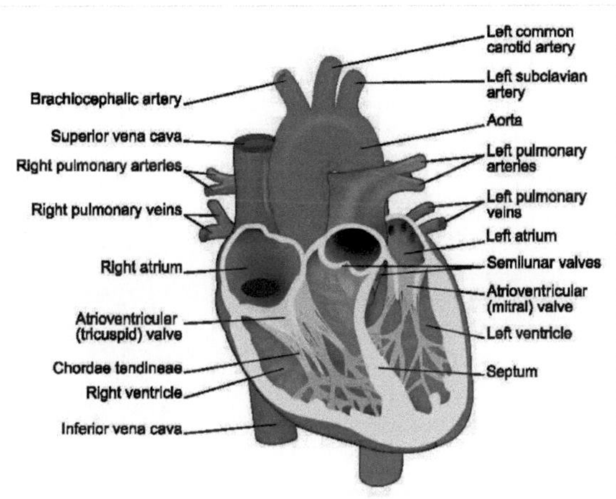

Structure diagram of the human heart from an anterior view. Blue components indicate de-oxygenated blood pathways and red components indicate oxygenated pathways.

and is composed of muscle which contracts. The inner layer is called the endocardium and is in contact with the blood that the heart pumps. Also, it merges with the inner lining (endothelium) of blood vessels and covers heart valves.[10]

The human heart has four chambers, two superior atria and two inferior ventricles. The atria are the receiving chambers and the ventricles are the discharging chambers. The pathway of blood through the human heart consists of a pulmonary circuit[11] and a systemic circuit. Deoxygenated blood flows through the heart in one direction, entering through the superior vena cava into the right atrium and is pumped through the tricuspid valve into the right ventricle before being pumped out through the pulmonary valve to the pulmonary arteries into the lungs. It returns from the lungs through the pulmonary veins to the left atrium where it is pumped through the mitral valve into the left ventricle before leaving through the aortic valve to the aorta.[12] [13]

In fish

Primitive fish have a four-chambered heart, but the chambers are arranged sequentially so that this primitive heart is quite unlike the four-chambered hearts of mammals and birds. The first chamber is the sinus venosus, which collects de-oxygenated blood, from the body, through the hepatic and cardinal veins. From here, blood flows into the atrium and then to the powerful muscular ventricle where the main pumping action will take place. The fourth and final chamber is the conus arteriosus which contains several valves and sends blood to the *ventral aorta*. The ventral aorta delivers blood to the gills where it is oxygenated and flows, through the dorsal aorta, into the rest of the body. (In tetrapods, the ventral aorta has divided in two; one half forms the ascending aorta, while the other forms the pulmonary artery).[8]

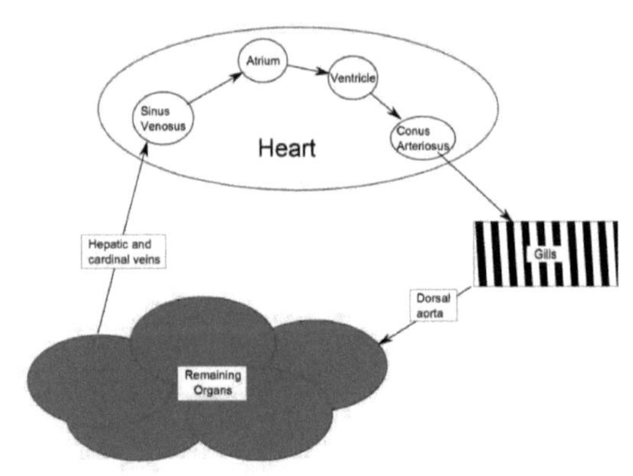

Schematic of simplified fish heart

In the adult fish, the four chambers are not arranged in a straight row but, instead form an S-shape with the latter two chambers lying above the former two. This relatively simpler pattern is found in cartilaginous fish and in the ray-finned fish. In teleosts, the conus arteriosus is very small and can more accurately be described as part of the aorta rather than of the heart proper. The conus arteriosus is not present in any amniotes, presumably having been absorbed into the ventricles over the course of evolution. Similarly, while the sinus venosus is present as a vestigial structure in some reptiles and birds, it is otherwise absorbed into the right atrium and is no longer distinguishable.[8]

In double circulatory systems

In amphibians and most reptiles, a double circulatory system is used but the heart is not completely separated into two pumps. The development of the double system is necessitated by the presence of lungs which deliver oxygenated blood directly to the heart.

In living amphibians, the atrium is divided into two separate chambers by the presence of a muscular septum even though there is only one ventricle. The sinus venosus, which remains large in amphibians but connects only to the right atrium, receives blood from the vena cavae, with the pulmonary vein by-passing it entirely to enter the left atrium.

In the heart of lungfish, the septum extends part-way into the ventricle. This allows for some degree of separation between the de-oxygenated bloodstream destined for the lungs and the oxygenated stream that is delivered to the rest of the body. The absence of such a division in living amphibian species may be at least partly due to the amount of respiration that occurs through the skin in such species; thus, the blood returned to the heart through the vena cavae is, in fact, already partially oxygenated. As a result, there may be less need for a finer division between the two bloodstreams than in lungfish or other tetrapods. Nonetheless, in at least some species of amphibian, the spongy nature of the ventricle seems to maintain more of a separation between the bloodstreams than appears the case at first glance. Furthermore, the conus arteriosus has lost its original valves and contains a spiral valve, instead, that divides it into two parallel parts, thus helping to keep the two bloodstreams separate.[8]

The heart of most reptiles (except for crocodilians; *see below*) has a similar structure to that of lungfish but, here, the septum is generally much larger. This divides the ventricle into two halves but, because the septum does not reach the whole length of the heart, there is a considerable gap near the openings to the pulmonary artery and the aorta. In practice, however, in the majority of reptilian species, there appears to be little, if any, mixing between the bloodstreams, so the aorta receives, essentially, only oxygenated blood.[8]

The fully divided heart

Archosaurs, (crocodilians, birds), and mammals show complete separation of the heart into two pumps for a total of four heart chambers; it is thought that the four-chambered heart of archosaurs evolved independently from that of mammals. In crocodilians, there is a small opening, the foramen of Panizza, at the base of the arterial trunks and there is some degree of mixing between the blood in each side of the heart; thus, only in birds and mammals are the two streams of blood – those to the pulmonary and systemic circulations – kept entirely separate by a physical barrier.[8]

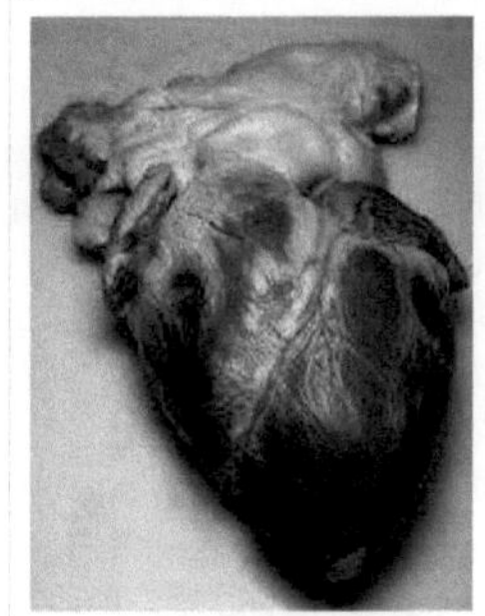

Human heart removed from a
64-year-old man

In the human body, the heart is usually situated in the middle of the thorax with the largest part of the heart slightly offset to the left, although sometimes it is on the right (see dextrocardia), underneath the sternum. The heart is usually felt to be on the left side because the left heart (left ventricle) is stronger (it pumps to all body parts). The left lung is smaller than the right lung because the heart occupies more of the left hemithorax. The heart is fed by the coronary circulation and is enclosed by a sac known as the pericardium; it is also surrounded by the lungs. The pericardium comprises two parts: the fibrous pericardium, made of dense fibrous connective tissue, and a double membrane structure (parietal and visceral pericardium) containing a serous fluid to reduce friction during heart contractions. The heart is located in the mediastinum, which is the central sub-division of the thoracic cavity. The mediastinum also contains other structures, such as the esophagus and trachea, and is flanked on either side by the right and left pulmonary cavities; these cavities house the lungs.[15]

The *apex* is the blunt point situated in an inferior (pointing down and left) direction. A stethoscope can be placed directly over the apex so that the beats can be counted. It is located posterior to the 5th intercostal space just medial of the left mid-clavicular line. In normal adults, the mass of the heart is 250–350 g (9–12 oz), or about twice the size of a clenched fist (it is about the size of a clenched fist in children), but an extremely diseased heart can be up to 1000 g (2 lb) in mass due to hypertrophy. It consists of four chambers, the two upper atria and the two lower ventricles.The heart is a myogenic muscular organ found in all animals with a circulatory system (including all vertebrates), that is responsible for pumping blood throughout the blood vessels by repeated, rhythmic contractions. The term cardiac (as in cardiology) means "related to the heart" and comes from the Greek καρδιά, kardia, for "heart". The vertebrate

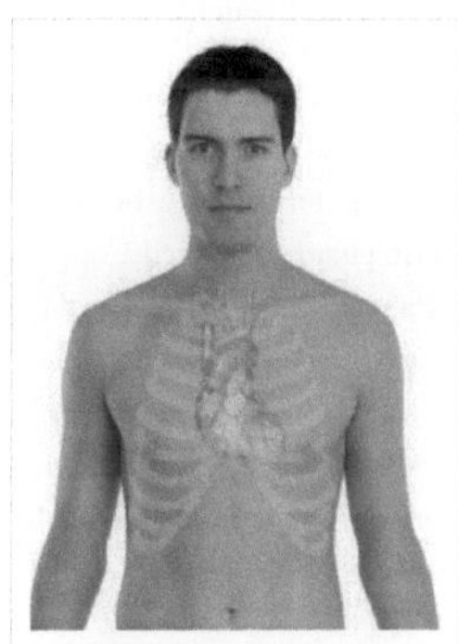

Surface anatomy of the human heart. The heart is demarcated by: -A point 9 cm to the left of the midsternal line (apex of the heart) -The seventh right sternocostal articulation -The upper border of the third right costal cartilage 1 cm from the right sternal line -The lower border of the second left costal cartilage 2.5 cm from the left lateral sternal line.[14]

heart is composed of cardiac muscle, which is an involuntary striated muscle tissue found only in this organ, and connective tissue. The average human heart, beating at 72 beats per minute, will beat approximately 2.5 billion times during an average 66 year lifespan. It weighs approximately 250 to 300 grams (9 to 11 oz) in females and 300 to 350 grams (11 to 12 oz) in males.[1] In invertebrates that possess a circulatory system, the heart is typically a tube or small sac and pumps fluid that contains water and nutrients such as proteins, fats, and sugars. In insects, the "heart" is often called the dorsal tube and insect "blood" is almost always not oxygenated since they usually respire (breathe) directly from their body surfaces (internal and external) to air. However, the hearts of some other arthropods (including spiders and crustaceans such as crabs and shrimp) and some other animals pump hemolymph, which contains the copper-based protein hemocyanin as an oxygen transporter similar to the iron-based hemoglobin in red blood cells found in vertebrates.

Functioning

In mammals, the function of the right side of the heart (see right heart) is to collect de-oxygenated blood, in the right atrium, from the body (via superior and inferior vena cavae) and pump it, through the tricuspid valve, via the right ventricle, into the lungs (pulmonary circulation) so that carbon dioxide can be dropped off and oxygen picked up (gas exchange). This happens through the passive process of diffusion. The left side (see left heart) collects oxygenated blood from the lungs into the left atrium. From the left atrium the blood moves to the left ventricle, through the bicuspid valve, which pumps it out to the body (via the aorta). On both sides, the lower ventricles are thicker and stronger than the upper atria. The muscle wall surrounding the left ventricle is thicker than the wall surrounding the right ventricle due to the higher force needed to pump the blood through the systemic circulation.

Starting in the right atrium, the blood flows through the tricuspid valve to the right ventricle. Here, it is pumped out the pulmonary semilunar valve and travels through the pulmonary artery to the lungs. From there, oxygenated blood flows back through the pulmonary vein to the left atrium. It then travels through the mitral valve to the left ventricle, from where it is pumped through the aortic semilunar valve to the aorta. The aorta forks and the blood is divided between major arteries which supply the upper and lower body. The blood travels in the arteries to the smaller arterioles and then, finally, to the tiny capillaries which feed each cell. The (relatively) deoxygenated blood then travels to the venules, which coalesce into veins, then to the inferior and superior venae cavae and finally back to the right atrium where the process began.

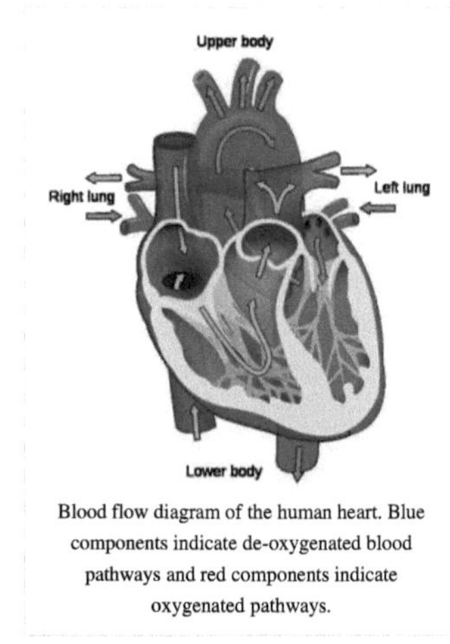

Blood flow diagram of the human heart. Blue components indicate de-oxygenated blood pathways and red components indicate oxygenated pathways.

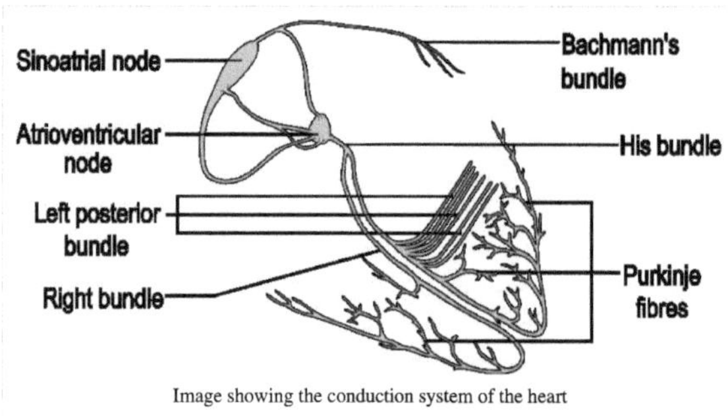

Image showing the conduction system of the heart

The heart is effectively a syncytium, a meshwork of cardiac muscle cells interconnected by contiguous cytoplasmic bridges. This relates to electrical stimulation of one cell spreading to neighboring cells.

Some cardiac cells are self-excitable, contracting without any signal from the nervous system, even if removed from the heart and placed in culture. Each of these cells have their own intrinsic contraction rhythm. A region of the human heart called the **sinoatrial (SA) node**, or pacemaker, sets the rate and timing at which all cardiac muscle cells contract. The SA node generates electrical impulses, much like those produced by nerve cells. Because cardiac muscle cells are electrically coupled by inter-calated disks between adjacent cells, impulses from the SA node spread rapidly through the walls of the artria, causing both artria to contract in unison. The impulses also pass to another region of specialized cardiac muscle tissue, a relay point called the **atrioventricular node**, located in the wall between the right atrium and the right ventricle. Here, the impulses are delayed for about 0.1s before spreading to the walls of the ventricle. The delay ensures that the artria empty completely before the ventricles contract. Specialized muscle fibers called Purkinje fibers then conduct the signals to the apex of the heart along and throughout the ventricular walls. The Purkinje fibres form conducting pathways called bundle branches. This entire cycle, a single heart beat, lasts about 0.8 seconds. The impulses generated during the heart cycle produce electrical currents, which are conducted through body fluids to the skin, where they can be detected by electrodes and recorded as an electrocardiogram (ECG or EKG).[16] The events related to the flow or blood pressure that occurs from the beginning of one heartbeat to the beginning of the next can be referred to a cardiac cycle. [17]

The SA node is found in all amniotes but not in more primitive vertebrates. In these animals, the muscles of the heart are relatively continuous and the sinus venosus coordinates the beat which passes in a wave through the remaining chambers. Indeed, since the sinus venosus is incorporated into the right atrium in amniotes, it is likely homologous with the SA node. In teleosts, with their vestigial sinus venosus, the main centre of coordination is, instead, in the atrium. The rate of heartbeat varies enormously between different species, ranging from around 20 beats per minute in codfish to around 600 in hummingbirds.[8]

Cardiac arrest is the sudden cessation of normal heart rhythm which can include a number of pathologies such as tachycardia, an extremely rapid heart beat which prevents the heart from effectively pumping blood, which is an irregular and ineffective heart rhythm, and asystole, which is the cessation of heart rhythm entirely.

Cardiac tamponade is a condition in which the fibrous sac surrounding the heart fills with excess fluid or blood, suppressing the heart's ability to beat properly. Tamponade is treated by pericardiocentesis, the gentle insertion of the needle of a syringe into the pericardial sac (avoiding the heart itself) on an angle, usually from just below the sternum, and gently withdrawing the tamponading fluids.

History of discoveries

The valves of the heart were discovered by a physician of the Hippocratean school around the 4th century BC, although their function was not fully understood. On dissection, arteries are typically empty of blood because of the fact that blood pools in the veins after death. Ancient anatomists subsequently assumed they were filled with air and served to transport it around the body.

Philosophers distinguished veins from arteries, but thought the pulse was a property of arteries themselves. Erasistratos observed that arteries cut during life bleed. He ascribed the fact to the phenomenon that air escaping from an artery is replaced with blood which entered by very small vessels between veins and arteries. Thus he apparently postulated capillaries, but with reversed flow of blood.

The Greek physician Galen (2nd century AD) knew blood vessels carried blood and identified venous (dark red) and arterial (brighter and thinner) blood, each with distinct and separate functions. Growth and energy were derived from venous blood created in the liver from chyle,

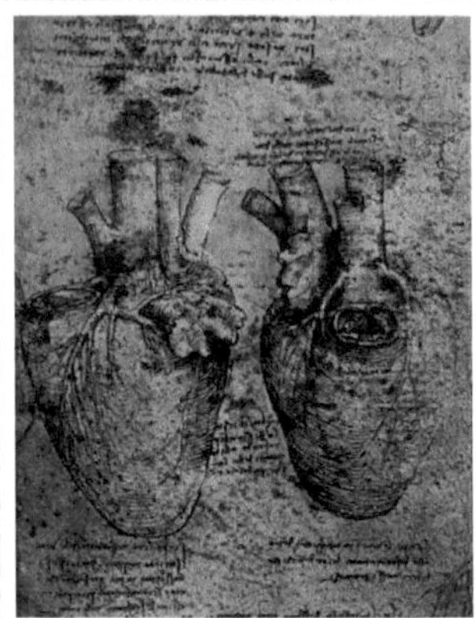

Heart and its blood vessels, by Leonardo da Vinci, 15th century

while arterial blood gave vitality by containing pneuma (air) and originated in the heart. Blood flowed from both creating organs to all parts of the body, where it was consumed and there was no return of blood to the heart or liver. The heart did not pump blood around, the heart's motion sucked blood in during diastole and the blood moved by the pulsation of the arteries themselves.

Galen believed the arterial blood was created by venous blood passing from the left ventricle to the right through 'pores' in the interventricular septum, while air passed from the lungs via the pulmonary artery to the left side of the heart. As the arterial blood was created, 'sooty' vapors were created and passed to the lungs, also via the pulmonary artery, to be exhaled.

For more recent technological developments, see Cardiac surgery.

See also

- Electrical conduction system of the heart
- Heart disease
- Langendorff Heart
- Physiology
- Trauma triad of death

References

[1] Kumar, Abbas, Fausto: *Robbins and Cotran Pathologic Basis of Disease*, 7th Ed. p. 556

[2] "Animal Tissues" (http://users.rcn.com/jkimball.ma.ultranet/BiologyPages/A/AnimalTissues.html). Users.rcn.com. 2010-08-13. . Retrieved 2010-10-17.

[3] "Main Frame Heart Development" (http://www.meddean.luc.edu/lumen/MedEd/GrossAnatomy/thorax0/heartdev/main_fra.html). Meddean.luc.edu. . Retrieved 2010-10-17.

[4] DuBose, Miller , Moutos. "Embryonic Heart Rates Compared in Assisted and Non-Assisted Pregnancies" (http://www.obgyn.net/us/us. asp?page=/us/cotm/0001/ehr2000). Obgyn.net. . Retrieved 2010-10-18..

[5] DuBose TJ, Cunyus JA, and Johnson L (1990). "Embryonic Heart Rate and Age". *J Diagn Med Sonography* **6**: 151–157. doi:10.1177/875647939000600306.

[6] DuBose, TJ (1996) *Fetal Sonography*, pp. 263–274; Philadelphia: WB Saunders ISBN 0-7216-5432-0

[7] Terry J. DuBose Sex, Heart Rate and Age (http://www.obgyn.net/english/pubs/features/dubose/ehr-age.htm)

[8]   Romer, Alfred Sherwood; Parsons, Thomas S. (1977). *The Vertebrate Body*. Philadelphia, PA: Holt-Saunders International. pp. 437–442. ISBN 0-03-910284-X.

[9]   MacDonald, Matthew (2009). *Your Body: The Missing Manual*. Sebastopol, CA: Pogue Press. ISBN 0-596-80174-2.

[10]   "Heart" (http://www.medicalook.com/human_anatomy/organs/Heart.html). *MedicaLook*. Medicalook.com. . Retrieved 2010-05-03.

[11]   "Pulmonary circuit" (http://medical-dictionary.thefreedictionary.com/Pulmonary+circuit). medical-dictionary.thefreedictionary.com. . Retrieved 2011-05-10.

[12]   Emergency Medical Responder 3rd Can Ed. Pearson, 2010 pp.131

[13]   Marieb, Elaine Nicpon. Human Anatomy & Physiology. 6th ed. Upper Saddle River: Pearson Education, 2003. Print

[14]   "Gray's Anatomy of the Human Body — 6. Surface Markings of the Thorax" (http://www.bartleby.com/107/284.html). Bartleby.com. . Retrieved 2010-10-18.

[15]   Maton, Anthea; Jean Hopkins, Charles William McLaughlin, Susan Johnson, Maryanna Quon Warner, David LaHart, Jill D. Wright (1993). *Human Biology and Health*. Englewood Cliffs, New Jersey: Prentice Hall. ISBN 0-13-981176-1. OCLC 32308337.

[16]   Campbell, Reece-Biology, 7th Ed. p.873,874

[17]   Guyton, A.C. & Hall, J.E. (2006) *Textbook of Medical Physiology* (11th ed.) Philadelphia: Elsevier Saunder ISBN 0-7216-0240-1

External links

- The Heart (http://www.bbc.co.uk/programmes/p003c1bh) on *In Our Time* at the BBC. (listen now (http://www.bbc.co.uk/iplayer/console/p003c1bh/In_Our_Time_The_Heart))
- Atlas of Human Cardiac Anatomy (http://www.vhlab.umn.edu/atlas/index.shtml) — Endoscopic views of beating hearts — Cardiac anatomy
- Heart contraction and blood flow (animation) (http://www.nhlbi.nih.gov/health/dci/Diseases/hhw/hhw_pumping.html)
- Heart Disease (http://www.heart.org.in/)
- eMedicine: Surgical anatomy of the heart (http://www.emedicine.com/ped/topic2902.htm)
- Animal hearts: fish, squid (http://users.rcn.com/jkimball.ma.ultranet/BiologyPages/A/AnimalHearts.html)
- Heart Information (http://www.pharmacyproductinfo.com/Heart.html)
- Oath of Awareness (http://www.oathofawareness.org/) Heart disease awareness site
- Dissection review of the anatomy of the Human Heart including vessels, internal and external features (http://anatomyguy.com/middle-mediastinum-and-heart-review/)
- Interactive 3D heart (http://thevirtualheart.org/anatomyindex.html) This realistic heart can be rotated, and all its components can be studied from any angle.
- Watch an animation explaining how the normal human heart works (http://www.heartfailurematters.org/EN/Animation/Pages/animation_1.aspx)

mrj:Йäнг

Pericarditis

Pericarditis	
Classification and external resources	
An ECG showing pericarditis. Note the ST elevation in multiple leads with slight reciprocal ST depression in aVR.	
ICD-10	I01.0 [1], I09.2 [2], I30 [3]-I32 [4]
ICD-9	420.0 [5], 420.90 [6], 420.91 [7], 420.99 [8], 423.1 [9], 423.2 [10]
DiseasesDB	9820 [11]
MedlinePlus	000182 [12]
eMedicine	med/1781 [13] emerg/412 [14]
MeSH	D010493 [15]

Pericarditis is an inflammation of the pericardium (the fibrous sac surrounding the heart). A characteristic chest pain is often present.

The causes of pericarditis are varied, including viral infections of the pericardium, idiopathic causes, uremic pericarditis, bacterial infections of the precardium (for i.e. *Mycobacterium tuberculosis*), post-infarct pericarditis (pericarditis due to heart attack), or Dressler's pericarditis.

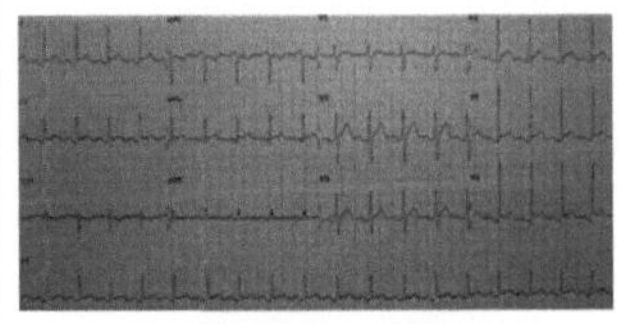

An ECG showing pericarditis.

Classification

Pericarditis can be classified according to the composition of the inflammatory exudate or in other words the composition of the fluid that accumulates around the heart.[16]

Types include:

- serous
- purulent
- fibrinous
- caseous
- hemorrhagic
- Post infarction

Acute vs. chronic

Depending on the time of presentation and duration, pericarditis is divided into "acute" and "chronic" forms. Acute pericarditis is more common than chronic pericarditis, and can occur as a complication of infections, immunologic conditions, or even as a result of a heart attack (myocardial infarction). Chronic pericarditis however is less common, a form of which is constrictive pericarditis. The following is the clinical classification of acute vs. chronic:

- *Clinically*: Acute (<6 weeks), Subacute (6 weeks to 6 months) and Chronic (>6 months)

Signs and symptoms

Substernal or left precordial pleuritic chest pain with radiation to the trapezius ridge (the bottom portion of scapula on the back), which is relieved by sitting up and bending forward and worsened by lying down (recumbent or supine position) or inspiration (taking a breath in), is the characteristic pain of pericarditis.[17] The pain may resemble the pain of angina pectoris or heart attack, but differs in that pain changes with body position, as opposed to heart attack pain that is pressure-like, and constant with radiation to the left arm and/or the jaw. Other symptoms of pericarditis may include dry cough, fever, fatigue, and anxiety. Due to similarity to myocardial infarction (heart attack) pain, pericarditis can be misdiagnosed as an acute myocardial infarction (a heart attack) solely based on the clinical data and so extreme suspicion on the part of the diagnostician is required. Ironically an acute myocardial infarction (heart attack) can also cause pericarditis, but often the presenting symptoms vary enough to warrant a diagnosis. The following table organises the clinical presentation of pericarditis:[17]

Characteristic/Parameter	Pericarditis	Myocardial infarction
Pain description	Sharp, pleuritic, retro-sternal (under the sternum) or left precordial (left chest) pain	Crushing, pressure-like, heavy pain. Described as "elephant on the chest."
Radiation	Pain radiates to the trapezius ridge (to the lowest portion of the scapula on the back) or no radiation.	Pain radiates to the jaw, or the left or arm, or does not radiate.
Exertion	Does not change the pain	Can increase the pain
Position	Pain is worse supine or upon inspiration (breathing in)	Not positional
Onset/duration	Sudden pain, that lasts for hours or sometimes days before a patient comes to the ER	Sudden or chronically worsening pain that can come and go in paroxysms or it can last for hours before the patient decides to come to the ER

Physical examinations

The classic sign of pericarditis is a friction rub auscultated on the cardiovascular examination usually on the lower left sternal border.[17] Other physical signs include a patient in distress, positional chest pain, diaphoresis (excessive sweating), and possibility of heart failure in form of precardial tamponade causing pulsus paradoxus, and the Beck's triad of hypotension (due to decreased cardiac output), distant (muffled) heart sounds, and JVD (jugular vein distention).

Acute complications

Pericarditis can progress to pericardial effusion and eventually cardiac tamponade. This can be seen in patients who are experiencing the classic signs of pericarditis but then show signs of relief, and progress to show signs of cardiac tamponade which include decreased alertness and lethargy, pulsus paradoxus (decrease of at least 10 mmHg of the systolic blood pressure upon inspiration), hypotension (due to decreased cardiac index), JVD (jugular vein distention from right sided heart failure and fluid overload), distant heart sounds on auscultation, and equilibration of all the diastolic blood pressures on cardiac catheterization due to the constriction of the pericardium by the fluid.

In such cases of cardiac tamponade, EKG or Holter monitor will then depict electrical alterans indicating wobbling of the heart in the fluid filled pericardium, and the capillary refill might decrease, as well as severe vascular collapse and altered mental status due to hypoperfusion of body organs by a heart that can not pump out blood effectively.

The diagnostic test for cardiac tamponade, is trans-esophageal echocardiography (TEE) although trans-thoracic echocardiography (TTE) can also be utilized in cases where there is a high suspicion of aortic dissection and high blood pressure, or in patients where esophageal probing is not feasible. Chest X-ray can depict a "water bottle" appearance of the heart in tamponade, although chest X-ray is not specific enough neither is it accurate enough in the acute setting. Of note is the fact that chest X-ray can be entirely normal in acute pericardial effusion/tamponade, so should not be relied upon as the sole diagnostic tool.

Causes

Infectious

Pericarditis may be caused by viral, bacterial, or fungal infection. The most common viral pathogen has traditionally been considered to be coxsackievirus based on studies in children from the 1960s, but recent data suggest that adults are most commonly affected with cytomegalovirus, herpesvirus, and HIV.[18] [19] Pneumococcus or tuberculous pericarditis are the most common bacterial forms. Anaerobic bacteria can also be rare cause.[20] Fungal pericarditis is usually due to histoplasmosis, or in immunocompromised hosts Aspergillus, Candida, and Coccidioides. The most common worldwide cause of pericarditis is infectious pericarditis with Tuberculosis.

Other

- Idiopathic: No identifiable etiology found after routine testing.
- Immunologic conditions including systemic lupus erythematosus (more common among women) or rheumatic fever
- Myocardial Infarction (Dressler's syndrome)
- Trauma to the heart, e.g. puncture, resulting in infection or inflammation
- Uremia (uremic pericarditis)
- Malignancy (as a paraneoplastic phenomenon)
- Side effect of some medications, e.g. isoniazid, cyclosporine, hydralazine, warfarin, and heparin
- Radiation induced
- Aortic dissection
- Tetracyclines
- Postpericardiotomy syndrome: Usually after CABG surgery

Laboratory tests

Laboratory values can show increased uric acid (BUN), or increased blood creatinine in cases of uremic pericarditis. Generally however, laboratory values are normal, but if there is a concurrent myocardial infarction (heart attack) or great stress to the heart, laboratory values may show increased cardiac markers like Troponin (I, T), CK-MB, Myoglobin, and LDH1 (Lactase Dehydrogenase isotype 1). The preferred intial diagnostic testing is the EKG which will show a 12-lead electrocardiogram with diffuse, non-specific, concave, ST segment-elevations all leads except aVR and V1[17] and PR segment-depression possible in any lead except aVR;[17] sinus tachycardia, and low-voltage QRS complexes can also be seen if there is subsymptomatic levels of pericardial effusion.

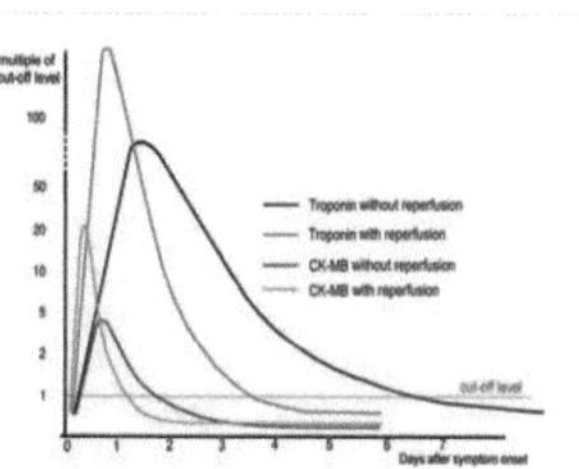

This diagram depicts the elevation of respective cardiac markers in a myocardial infarction (heart attack). Although this diagram is only for heart attack, elevated values of these markers might be seen in pericarditis.

Since the mid-19th Century, retrospective diagnosis of pericarditis has been made upon the finding of adhesions of the pericardium.[21] When pericarditis is diagnosed clinically, the underlying cause is often never known; it may be discovered in only 16[22] to 22[23] percent of patients with acute pericarditis.

Treatment

The treatment in viral or idiopathic pericarditis is with Aspirin,[17] or non-steroidal anti-inflammatory drugs (NSAIDs such as naproxen). Severe cases may require:

- pericardiocentesis to treat pericardial effusion/tamponade
- antibiotics to treat tuberculosis or other bacterial causes.
- steroids are used in acute pericarditis but are not favored because they increase chance of recurrent pericarditis.
- colchicine is a very effective treatment option. If Aspirin and NSAIDs are not sufficient, colchicine should be added to the regimen.
- in rare cases, surgery
- in cases of contrictive pericarditis, pericardectomy

References

[1] http://apps.who.int/classifications/icd10/browse/2010/en#/I01.0

[2] http://apps.who.int/classifications/icd10/browse/2010/en#/I09.2

[3] http://apps.who.int/classifications/icd10/browse/2010/en#/I30

[4] http://apps.who.int/classifications/icd10/browse/2010/en#/I32

[5] http://www.icd9data.com/getICD9Code.ashx?icd9=420.0

[6] http://www.icd9data.com/getICD9Code.ashx?icd9=420.90

[7] http://www.icd9data.com/getICD9Code.ashx?icd9=420.91

[8] http://www.icd9data.com/getICD9Code.ashx?icd9=420.99

[9] http://www.icd9data.com/getICD9Code.ashx?icd9=423.1

[10] http://www.icd9data.com/getICD9Code.ashx?icd9=423.2

[11] http://www.diseasesdatabase.com/ddb9820.htm

[12] http://www.nlm.nih.gov/medlineplus/ency/article/000182.htm

[13] http://www.emedicine.com/med/topic1781.htm

[14] http://www.emedicine.com/emerg/topic412.htm#

[15] http://www.nlm.nih.gov/cgi/mesh/2011/MB_cgi?field=uid&term=D010493

[16] images (http://library.med.utah.edu/WebPath/CVHTML/CVIDX.html)

[17] American College of Physicians (ACP). "Pericardial disease" (http://www.acponline.org/products_services/mksap/15/complete.htm). *Medical Knowledge Self-Assessment Program (MKSAP-15): Cardiovascular Medicine.* p. 64. ISBN 978-934465-28-8. .

[18] AU Corey GR; Campbell PT; Van Trigt P; Kenney RT; O'Connor CM; Sheikh KH; Kisslo JA; Wall TC (August 1993). "Etiology of large
     pericardial effusions". *American Journal of Medicine* **95** (2): 209–13. doi:10.1016/0002-9343(93)90262-N. PMID 8356985.

[19] Campbell PT; Li JS; Wall TC; O'Connor CM; Van Trigt P; Kenney RT; Melhus O; Corey GR (April 1995). "Cytomegalovirus pericarditis:
     a case series and review of the literature". *American Journal of Medical Science* **309** (4): 229–34. doi:10.1097/00000441-199504000-00009.
     PMID 7900747.

[20] Brook I. Pericarditis caused by anaerobic bacteria.Int J Antimicrob Agents 2009; 297-300.

[21] Austin Flint (1862). "Lectures on the diagnosis of diseases of the heart: Lecture VIII". *American Medical Times: Being a weekly series of the
     New York Journal of Medicine* **5** (July to December): 309–311.

[22] Permanyer-Miralda G; Sagrista-Sauleda J; Soler-Soler J (October 1, 1985). "Primary acute pericardial disease: a prospective series of 231
     consecutive patients". *American Journal of Cardiology* **56** (10): 623–30. doi:10.1016/0002-9149(85)91023-9. PMID 4050698.

[23] Zayas R; Anguita M; Torres F; Gimenez D; Bergillos F; Ruiz M; Ciudad M; Gallardo A; Valles F (February 15, 1995). "Incidence of
     specific etiology and role of methods for specific etiologic diagnosis of primary acute pericarditis". *American Journal of Cardiology* **75** (5):
     378–82. doi:10.1016/S0002-9149(99)80558-X. PMID 7856532.

General References

- Troughton RW, Asher CR, Klein AL (February 2004). "Pericarditis" (http://linkinghub.elsevier.com/retrieve/
  pii/S0140-6736(04)15648-1). *Lancet* **363** (9410): 717–27. doi:10.1016/S0140-6736(04)15648-1.
  PMID 15001332.

- Maisch B, Seferović PM, Ristić AD, *et al.* (April 2004). "Guidelines on the diagnosis and management of
  pericardial diseases executive summary; The Task force on the diagnosis and management of pericardial diseases
  of the European society of cardiology" (http://eurheartj.oxfordjournals.org/cgi/content/full/25/7/587). *Eur.
  Heart J.* **25** (7): 587–610. doi:10.1016/j.ehj.2004.02.002. PMID 15120056.

External links

- Pericarditis — Cleveland Clinic (http://my.clevelandclinic.org/heart/disorders/other/pericarditis.aspx)
- Pericarditis — National Library of Medicine (http://www.nlm.nih.gov/medlineplus/ency/article/000182.
  htm)
- Pericarditis — National Heart Lung Blood Institute (http://www.nhlbi.nih.gov/health/dci/Diseases/peri/
  peri_whatis.html)

Differential_diagnosis

Differential diagnosis	
Intervention	
MeSH	D003937 [1]

A **differential diagnosis** (sometimes abbreviated **DDx, ddx, DD, D/Dx**, or $\Delta\Delta$) is a systematic diagnostic method used to identify the presence of an entity where multiple alternatives are possible (and the process may be termed **differential diagnostic procedure**), and may also refer to any of the included candidate alternatives (which may also be termed **candidate condition**). This method is essentially a process of elimination, or at least, rendering of the probabilities of candidate conditions to negligible levels. In this sense, probabilities are, in fact, imaginative parameters in the mind or hardware of the diagnostician or system, while in reality the target (such as a patient) either has a condition or not with an actual probability of either 0 or 100%.

Differential diagnostic procedures are used by physicians, psychiatrists, and other trained medical professionals to diagnose the specific disease in a patient, or, at least, to eliminate any imminently life-threatening conditions.

Differential diagnosis can be regarded as implementing aspects of the hypothetico-deductive method in the sense that the potential presence of candidate diseases or conditions can be viewed as hypotheses which are further processed as being true or false.

General components

There are various methods of performing a differential diagnostic procedure, but in general, it is based on the idea that one begins by considering the most common diagnosis first: a head cold versus meningitis, for example. As a reminder, medical students are taught the adage, "When you hear hoofbeats, look for horses, not zebras," which means look for the simplest, most common explanation first. Only after the simplest diagnosis has been ruled out should the clinician consider more complex or exotic diagnoses.

A differential diagnostic procedure can be performed by that the doctor first gathers all information about the patient and create a symptoms list. The list can be in writing or in the doctor's head, as long as he or she makes a list. Second, the doctor should make a list of all possible causes (also termed "candidate conditions") of the symptoms. Again, this can be in writing or in the doctor's head but it must be done. Third, the doctor should prioritize the list by placing the most urgently dangerous possible cause of the symptoms at the top of the list. Fourth, the doctor should rule out or treat the possible causes beginning with the most urgently dangerous condition and working his or her way down the list. "Rule out" practically means to use tests and other scientific methods to render a condition of clinically negligible probability of being the cause.

In some cases, there will remain *no* diagnosis; this suggests the physician has made an error, or that the true diagnosis is unknown to medicine. Removing diagnoses from the list is done by making observations and using tests that should have different results, depending on which diagnosis is correct.

Mnemonics are routinely taught to medical students to ensure that all possible pathological processes are considered, for example *VINDICATE*: **V**ascular, **I**nflammatory, **N**eoplastic, **D**egenerative/Deficiency, **I**diopathic/Intoxication, **C**ongenital, **A**utoimmune/Allergic, **T**raumatic, **E**ndocrine[2]

Specific methods

There are several methods for performing a differential diagnostic procedure, and several variants among those in turn. Furthermore, a differential diagnostic procedure can be used concomitantly or switchingly with protocols, guidelines or other diagnostic procedures (such as pattern-recognition or using medical algorithms).

For example, in case of medical emergency, there may not be enough time to do any detailed calculations or estimations of different probabilities, in which case the ABC protocol may be more appropriate. At a later, less acute, situation, there may be a switch to a more comprehensive differential diagnostic procedure.

The differential diagnostic procedure may be easier in the finding of a *pathognomonic* sign or symptom, in which it is almost certain that the target condition is present, and in the absence of finding a *sine qua non* sign or symptom, in which case it is almost certain that the target condition is absent. In reality, however, the subjective probability of the presence of a condition is never exactly 100% or 0%, so in reality the procedure is usually aimed at specifying the various probabilities in order to form indications for further actions.

By epidemiology

One method of performing a differential diagnosis by epidemiology aims to estimate the probability of each candidate condition by comparing their probabilities to have occurred in the first place in the individual. It is based on probabilities related both to the presentation (such as pain) and probabilities of the various candidate conditions (such as diseases).

Theory

The probability that a presentation or condition would have occurred in the first place in an individual is not same as the probability that the presentation or condition *has* occurred in the individual, because the presentation *has* occurred by 100% certainty in the individual. Yet, the contributive probability fractions of each condition are assumed to be the same, relatively:

, where:

- *P(Presentation is caused by condition in individual)* is the probability that the presentation is caused by condition in the individual
- *condition* without further specification refers to any candidate condition
- *P(Presentation has occurred in individual)* is the probability that the presentation has occurred in the individual, which is 100%
- *P(Presentation WHOIFPI by condition)* is the probability that the presentation Would Have Occurred In the First Place in the Individual by condition
- *P(Presentation WHOIFPI)* is the probability that the presentation Would Have Occurred In the First Place in the Individual

P(Presentation has occurred in individual) is 100% and can therefore be replaced by 1, and can be ignored since division by 1 does not make any difference:

The total probability of the presentation to have occurred in the individual can be approximated as the sum of the individual candidate conditions:

Also, the probability of the presentation to have been caused by any candidate condition is proportional to the probability of the condition, depending on what rate it causes the presentation:

, where:

- *P(Presentation WHOIFPI by condition)* is the probability that the presentation Would Have Occurred In the First Place in the Individual by condition
- *P(Condition WHOIFPI)* is the probability that the condition Would Have Occurred In the First Place in the Individual

- $r_{Condition \rightarrow presentation}$ is the rate for which condition causes the presentation, that is, the fraction of people with condition that manifest with the presentation

The probability that a condition would have occurred in the first place in an individual is approximately equal to that of a population that is as similar to the individual as possible except for the current presentation, compensated where possible by relative risks given by known risk factor that distinguish the individual from the population:

, where:

- *P(Condition WHOIFPI)* is the probability that the condition Would Have Occurred In the First Place in the Individual
- $RR_{condition}$ is the relative risk for condition conferred by known risk factors in the individual that are not present in the population
- *P(Condition in population) is the probability that the condition occurs in a population that is as similar to the individual as possible except for the presentation*

The following table demonstrates how these relations can be made for a series of candidate conditions:

	Candidate condition 1	Candidate condition 2	Candidate condition 3
P(Condition in population)	*P(Condition 1 in population)*	*P(Condition 2 in population)*	*P(Condition 3 in population)*
$RR_{condition}$	RR_1	RR_2	RR_3
P(Condition WHOIFPI)	*P(Condition 1 WHOIFPI)*	*P(Condition 2 WHOIFPI)*	*P(Condition 3 WHOIFPI)*
$r_{Condition \rightarrow presentation}$	$r_{Condition\ 1 \rightarrow presentation}$	$r_{Condition\ 2 \rightarrow presentation}$	$r_{Condition\ 3 \rightarrow presentation}$
P(Presentation WHOIFPI by condition)	*P(Presentation WHOIFPI by condition 1)*	*P(Presentation WHOIFPI by condition 2)*	*P(Presentation WHOIFPI by condition 3)*
P(Presentation WHOIFPI) = the sum of the probabilities in row just above			
P(Presentation is caused by condition in individual)	P(Presentation is caused by condition 1 in individual)	P(Presentation is caused by condition 2 in individual)	P(Presentation is caused by condition 3 in individual)

One additional "candidate condition" is the instance of there being no abnormality, and the presentation is only a (usually relatively unlikely) appearance of a basically normal state. Its probability in the population (*P(No abnormality in population)*) is complementary to the sum of probabilities of "abnormal" candidate conditions.

Example

This example case is made to demonstrate how this method may be applied, but does not intend to be a guideline for handling similar cases in reality. Also, the example uses relatively specified numbers with sometimes several decimals, while in reality there are often simply rough estimations, such as of likelihoods being "very high", "high", "low" or "very low", but still using the general principles of the method.

For an individual (who becomes the "patient" in this example), a blood test of, for example, serum calcium shows a result just above the standard reference range, which, by most definitions, classifies as hypercalcemia, which becomes the "presentation" in this case. A physician (who becomes the "diagnostician" in this example), who does not currently see the patient, gets to know about his finding.

By practical reasons, the physician considers that there is enough test indication to have a look at the patient's medical records. For simplicity, let's say that the only information given in the medical records is a family history of primary hyperparathyroidism (here abbreviated as PH), which may explain the finding of hypercalcemia. For this patient, let's say that the resultant hereditary risk factor is estimated to confer a relative risk of 10 ($RR_{PH} = 10$).

The physician considers that there is enough motivation to perform a differential diagnostic procedure for the finding of hypercalcemia. The main causes of hypercalcemia are primary hyperparathyroidism (PH) and cancer, so for simplicity, the list of candidate conditions that the physician could think of can be given as:

- Primary hyperparathyroidism (PH)
- Cancer
- Other diseases that the physician could think of (which is simply termed "other conditions" for the rest of this example)
- No disease (or no abnormality), and the finding is caused entirely by statistical variability

The the probability that **primary hyperparathyroidism** (PH) would have occurred in the first place in the individual ($P(PH\ WHOIFPI)$) can be calculated as follows:

Let's say that the last blood test taken by the patient was half a year ago and was normal, and that the incidence of primary hyperparathyroidism in a general population that appropriately matches the individual (except for the presentation and mentioned heredity) is 1 in 4000 per year. Ignoring more detailed retrospective analyses (such as including speed of disease progress and lag time of medical diagnosis), the time-at-risk for having developed primary hyperparathyroidism can roughly be regarded as being the last half year, because a previously developed hypercalcemia would probably have been caught up by the previous blood test. This corresponds to a probability of primary hyperparathyroidism (PH) in the population of:

With the relative risk conferred from the family history, the probability that primary hyperparathyroidism (PH) would have occurred in the first place in the individual given from the currently available information becomes:

Primary hyperparathyroidism can be assumed to cause hypercalcemia in essentially 100% of the time ($r_{PH\ \&rarr\ hypercalcemia} = 1$), so this independently calculated probability of primary hyperparathyroidism (PH) can be assumed to be the same as the probability of being a cause of the presentation:

For **cancer**, the same time-at-risk is assumed for simplicity, and let's say that the incidence of cancer in the area is estimated at 1 in 250 per year, giving an population probability of cancer of:

For simplicity, let's say that any association between a family history of primary hyperparathyroidism and risk of cancer is ignored, so the relative risk for the individual to have contracted cancer in the first place is similar to that of the population ($RR_{cancer} = 1$):

However, hypercalcemia only occurs in, very approximately, 10% of cancers,[3] ($r_{cancer\ \&rarr\ hypercalcemia} = 0.1$), so:

The probabilities that hypercalcemia would have occurred in the first place by other candidate conditions can be calculated in a similar manner. However, for simplicity, let's say that that the probability that any of these would have occurred in the first place is calculated to be 0.0005 in this example.

For the instance of there being **no disease**, the corresponding probability in the population is complementary to the sum of probabilities for other conditions:

The probability that the individual would be healthy in the first place can be assumed to be the same:

The rate at which the case of no abnormal condition still ends up in a measurement of serum calcium of being above the standard reference range (thereby classifying as hypercalcemia) is, by the definition of standard reference range, less than 2.5%. However, this probability can be further specified by considering how much the measurement deviates from the mean in the standard reference range. Let's say that the serum calcium measurement was 1.30 mmol/L, which, with a standard reference range established at 1.05 to 1.25 mmol/L, corresponds to a standard score of 3 and a corresponding probability of 0.14% that such degree of hypercalcemia would have occurred in the first place in the case of no abnormality:

Subsequently, the probability that hypercalemia would have resulted from no disease can be calculated as:

The probability that hypercalcemia would have occurred in the first place in the individual can thus be calculated as:

Subsequently, the probability that hypercalcemia is caused by primary hyperparathyroidism (PH) in the individual can be calculated as:

Similarly, the probability that hypercalcemia is caused by cancer in the individual can be calculated as:

, and for other candidate conditions:

, and the probability that there actually is no disease:

For clarification, these calculations are given as the table in the method description:

	PH	Cancer	Other conditions	No disease
P(Condition in population)	0.000125	0.002	-	0.997
RR_x	10	1	-	-
P(Condition WHOIFPI)	0.00125	0.002	-	-
$r_{Condition \rightarrow hypercalcemia}$	1	0.1	-	0.0014
P(hypercalcemia WHOIFPI by condition)	0.00125	0.0002	0.0005	0.0014
P(hypercalcemia WHOIFPI) = 0.00335				
P(hypercalcemia is caused by condition in individual)	37.3%	6.0%	14.9%	41.8%

Thus, this method estimates that the probabilities that the hypercalcemia is caused by primary hyperparathyroidism, cancer, other conditions or no disease at all are 37.3%, 6.0%, 14.9% and 41.8%, respectively, which may be used in estimating further test indications.

This case is continued in the example of the method described in the next section.

By independently and profile-relative probabilities

The procedure of differential diagnosis can become extremely complex if it would fully take additional tests and treatments into consideration. One method that is somewhat a tradeoff between being clinically perfect and being relatively simple to calculate is one that assigns two kinds of likelihood parameters for each disease or other condition that is included in the list of differential diagnoses; one independently calculated odds in favor of the condition, and one probability that is relative to the entire profile of conditions and their odds respectively.

Theory

For each candidate condition, this method first estimates an independently calculated *odds in favor*, which initially corresponds to the probability that the individual would have developed the condition in the first place, as used in the previously mentioned method using epidemiology. If previously calculated as a probability, it can be converted to *odds in favor* by:

These independently calculated odds in favor, in the format of their value *to one*, are summed together in this method, and the resultant value is be used to estimate a profile-relative probability for each candidate condition, as follows:

, where:

- $PRP_{condition}$ is the profile-relative probability of a condition
- $ICO_{condition}$ is the independently calculated odds in favor of a condition as a cause of the presentation
- ICO_{all} is the sum of all independently calculated odds in favor, of all candidate conditions

The profile-relative probabilities correspond to the probabilities of each condition of causing the presentation (*P(Presentation is caused by condition in individual)*), and are more clinically useful than the individually calculated odds, similarly to that the probabilities of conditions having occurred are more clinically useful than that the conditions would have occurred in the first place as mentioned in the epidemiology-based method. Therefore, it is the profile-relative probabilities that are used for estimating the indications for further medical tests, treatments or other actions in this method.

If there is an indication for a test, and it returns with a result, then the procedure is repeated by making new estimations of independently calculated odds for candidate conditions where they have likely changed, in turn likely resulting in a different sum of all independently calculated odds, and thereby different profile-relative probabilities.

With different profile-relative probabilities, the indications for further tests, treatments or other actions have changed as well, and are therefore estimated anew, and so the procedure can be repeated until an *end point* where there no longer is any indication for currently performing further actions. Such an end point mainly occurs when one candidate condition becomes so certain that no test can be found that is powerful enough to change the relative probability-profile enough to motivate any current change in further actions. Tactics for reaching such an end point with as few tests as possible includes making tests with high specificity for conditions of already outstandingly high profile-relative probability, because the high likelihood ratio positive for such tests is very high, bringing all less likely conditions to relatively lower probabilities. Alternatively, tests with high sensitivity for competing candidate conditions, such tests have a high likelihood ratio negative, potentially bringing the probabilities for competing candidate conditions to negligible levels. If such negligible probabilities are achieved, these conditions can be decided to be *ruled out*, and the differential diagnostic procedure continues with only the remaining candidate conditions.

Comparing to the previously mentioned epidemiology-based method, this method can be used with much more ease for including additional tests. However, this method is not so good at establishing initial probabilities, but can, on the other hand, be a good complementing method upon which to continue previously calculated probabilities from, for example, an epidemiology-based method.

Example

This example continues for the same patient as in the example for the epidemiology-based method. As with the previous example of epidemiology-based method, this example case is made to demonstrate how this method may be applied, but does not intend to be a guideline for handling similar cases in reality. Also, the example uses relatively specified numbers, while in reality there are often just rough estimations.

The probabilities that the presentation would have occurred in the first place for each condition ("P(Presentation WHOIFPI by condition) *can initially be set as the individually calculated probabilities, and the resultant probabilities of each condition of causing the presentation can initially be set as the profile relative probabilities:*

	PH	Cancer	Other conditions	No disease
Independently calculated probability (ICP)	0.00125	0.0002	0.0005	0.0014
Profile-relative probability (PRP)	37.3%	6.0%	14.9%	41.8%

The condition of highest profile-relative probability (except "no disease") is primary hyperparathyroidism (PH), but cancer is still of major concern, because if it is the actual causative condition for the hypercalcemia, then the choice of whether to treat or not likely means life or death for the patient, in effect potentially putting the indication at a similar level for further tests for both of these conditions. Because the

Here, let's say that the physician considers the profile-relative probabilities of being of enough concern to indicate to send the patient a call for a doctor's visit, with an additional visit to the medical laboratory for an additional blood test complemented with further analyses, including parathyroid hormone for the suspicion of primary hyperparathyroidism.

For simplicity, let's say that the doctor first receives the result for the parathyroid hormone analysis, and that it showed a parathyroid hormone level that is elevated relatively to what would be expected by the calcium level.

Such a constellation can be estimated to have a sensitivity of approximately 70% and a specificity of approximately 90% for primary hyperparathyroidism. [4] This confers a likelihood ratio positive of 7 for primary hyperparathyroidism.

The target value in this method is the independently calculated odds in favor of primary hyperparathyroidism, denoted *Pre-CaP* because it corresponds to before (Latin preposition *prae* means before) the calcium- and parathyroid hormone related test.

, where:

- $PreCaP\ ICO_{PH}$ is the independently calculated odds in favor of primary hyperparathyroidism before the calcium and parathyroid hormone related test
- ICP_{PH} is the independently calculated probability for primary hyperparathyroidism before the calcium and parathyroid hormone related test, previously given as 0.00125, resulting in:

Here, the difference between odds and probability is negligible because the value is very low.

The same can be done for the other candidate conditions, also resulting in negligible differences between odds and probabilities (although such differences can be substantial at higher values):

	PH	Cancer	Other conditions	No disease
Independently calculated probability (ICP)	0.00125	0.0002	0.0005	0.0014
Pre-CaP ICO	0.00125	0.0002	0.0005	0.0014

With the likelihood ratio positive of 7 for the calcium- and parathyroid hormone related test, the post-test odds is calculated as:

, where:

- $PostCaP\ ICO_{PH}$ is the independently calculated odds for primary hyperparathyroidism after the calcium and parathyroid hormone related test, given at 0.00125
- $PreCaP\ ICO_{PH}$ is the independently calculated odds in favor of primary hyperparathyroidism before the calcium and parathyroid hormone related test
- $LH+$ is the likelihood ratio positive for the test

Subsequently, the sum of all independently calculated odds after the calcium- and parathyroid hormone related test becomes:

The profile-relative probability for primary hyperparathyroidism (PH) after this test is calculated as:

, where:

- $PostCaP\ PRP_{PH}$ is the profile-relative probability for primary hyperparathyroidism after the calcium and parathyroid hormone related test
- $PostCaP\ ICO_{all}$ is the sum of all independently calculated odds after the calcium- and parathyroid hormone related test
- $PostCaP\ ICO_{PH}$ is the independently calculated odds for primary hyperparathyroidism after the calcium and parathyroid hormone related test

These are calculated similarly for the other conditions, but in this case with independently calculated post-test odds being same as pre-test odds, resulting as:

	PH	Cancer	Other conditions	No disease
PostCaP ICO	0.00875	0.0002	0.0005	0.0014
PostCaP PRP	80.6%	1.8%	4.6%	12.9%

These "new" percentages, including a profile-relative probability of 80% for primary hyperparathyroidism, underlie any indications for further tests, treatments or other actions. In this case, let's say that the physician continues the plan for the patient to attend a doctor's visit for further checkup, especially focused at primary hyperparathyroidism.

A doctor's visit can, theoretically, be regarded as a series of tests, including both questions in a medical history and components of a physical examination, where the post-test probability of a previous test can be used as the pre-test probability of the next. The indications for choosing the next test is dynamically influenced by the results of previous tests.

Let's say that the patient in this example is revealed to have depression, bone pain, joint pain and constipation of more severerity than what would be expected by the hypercalcemia itself, supporting the suspicion of primary hyperparathyroidism,[5] and let's say that the likelihood ratios for the tests, when multiplied together, roughly results in a product of 10 for primary hyperparathyroidism.

All the tests of the history and examination can concomitantly be used to estimate likelihood ratios for the presence of cancer, and let's say that the product of the likelihood ratios is estimated to be 3.

Tests for other conditions were basically all negative, and let's say that the resultant probability after the history and examination becomes 0.0005.

Continuing from the calcium- and parathyroid hormone related test, its post-test independently calculated odds are used as pre-test independently calculated odds for the medical history and physical examination (here abbreviated as H&E), with the ensuing calculations following the same overall pattern as the previous calcium- and parathyroid hormone related test:

	PH	Cancer	Other conditions	No disease
PreH&E ICO	0.00875	0.0002	0.0005	0.0014
Likelihood ratio by H&E	10	3	-	-
PostH&E ICO	0.0875	0.0006	0.0005	0.0014
PostH&E ICO$_{all}$	0.09			
PostH&E PRP	97.2%	0.7%	0.6%	1.6%

These profile relative probabilities after the history and examination may make the physician confident enough to plan the patient for surgery for a parathyroidectomy to resect the affected tissue.

At this point, the profile-relative probability of "other conditions" is so low that the physician cannot think of any test for them that could make a difference that would be substantial enough to form an indication for such a test, and the physician thereby regards "other conditions" as ruled out, in this case not primarily by specific test for such other conditions that were negative, but rather by the absence of positive tests so far.

For "cancer", the cutoff at which to confidently regard it as ruled out may be more stringent because of severe consequences of missing it, so the physician may consider that at least a histopathologic examination of the resected tissue is indicated.

This case is continued in the example of *Combinations* in corresponding section below.

Finding candidate conditions

The validity of both methods described above are dependent of inclusion of candidate conditions that are responsible for as large part as possible of the probability of having developed the condition, and it's clinically important to include those where relatively fast initiation of therapy is most likely to result in greatest benefit. The need to find more candidate conditions for inclusion increases with increasing severity of the presentation itself. For example, if the only presentation is a deviating laboratory parameter and all common harmful underlying conditions have been ruled out, then it may be acceptable to stop finding more candidate conditions, but this would much more likely be unacceptable if the presentation would have been severe pain.

Combinations

If two conditions appear as certain by their independently calculated probabilities, then there is a strong indication that the condition is a combination of the two, which can be added to the list of candidate conditions and be calculated independently for further evaluation.

To continue the example used in independently and profile-relative probabilities, let's say that the ensuing surgery and histopathologic examination of the resected tissue confirms primary hyperparathyroidism, having a very high specificity, and let's say that it gives a likelihood ratio of 1000 in this case. However, let's also say that the histopathologic examination also showed a malignant pattern, and let's say that this pattern gives a likelihood ratio for cancer of 1000 as well. The resultant independently calculated odds in favor of primary hyperparathyroidism and cancer become 87.5 and 0.6, respectively, with profile-relative probabilities of 99.3% and 0.7%, respectively. However, at this point, the individually calculated odds in favor of cancer of 0.6, corresponding to an individually calculated probability of 37.5%, are high enough to consider that the patient actually has a combination of primary hyperparathyroidism and cancer, that is, in this case, parathyroid carcinoma. To evaluate its possibility by this method, the combination can be added to the list of candidate conditions, followed by processing by every relevant test performed so far. By an initial method by epidemiology, the incidence of parathyroid carcinoma is estimated at about 1 in 6 million people per year,[6] giving a very low probability before taking any tests into consideration. Still, the probability that a non-malignant primary hyperparathyroidism would have occurred at the same time as an unrelated non-carcinoma cancer that presents with malignant cells in the parathyroid gland is calculated by multiplying the probabilities of the two, resulting in a negligible probability in comparison. So, focusing on parathyroid carcinoma, let's say that a review in regard to the subsequent blood tests, medical history, physical examination, surgery observations and histopathological examination result in rather high likelihood ratios, in turn resulting in a profile-relative probability high enough for an indication for making a confirmatory test for parathyroid cancer. In reality, the histopathologist may have recognized parathyroid carcinoma by pattern-recognition directly and, with or without specific tissue processing, may have given a certain diagnostic opinion of parathyroid carcinoma.

Let's finally say that the diagnosis of parathyroid carcinoma resulted in an extended surgery that removed remaining malignant tissue before it had metastasized, and the patient lived happily ever after.

Machine differential diagnosis

Further information: Clinical decision support system

Machine differential diagnosis is the use of computer software to partly or fully make a differential diagnosis. It may be regarded as an application of artificial intelligence.

Many studies demonstrate improvement of quality of care and reduction of medical errors by using such decision support systems. Some of these systems are designed for a specific medical problem such as schizophrenia,[7] Lyme disease[8] or ventilator-associated pneumonia.[9] Others such as Iliad, QMR, DiagnosisPro,[10] and VisualDx [11] are designed to cover all major clinical and diagnostic findings to assist physicians with faster and more accurate diagnosis.

However, these tools all still require advanced medical skills in order to rate the symptoms and choose additional tests to deduce the probabilities of different diagnoses. Thus, non-professionals still need to see a health care provider in order to get a proper diagnosis.

History

The method of differential diagnosis was first suggested for use in the diagnosis of mental disorders by Emil Kraepelin. It is more systematic than the old-fashioned method of diagnosis by *gestalt* (impression).

Alternative medical meanings

Differential diagnosis is also used more loosely, to refer simply to a list of the most common causes of a given symptom, to a list of disorders similar to a given disorder, or to such lists when they are annotated with advice on how to narrow the list down (the book *French's Index of Differential Diagnosis*, ISBN 0340810475, is an example). Thus, a differential diagnosis in this sense is medical information specially organized to aid in diagnosis.

Usage apart from in medicine

Methods similar to those of differential diagnostic processes in medicine are also is used by biological taxonomists to identify and classify organisms, living and extinct. For example, after finding an unknown species, there can first be a listing of all potential species, followed by ruling out of one by one until, optimally, only one potential choice remains.

See also

- List of medical symptoms
- Diagnosis of exclusion
- Comorbidity
- Dual diagnosis

References

[1] http://www.nlm.nih.gov/cgi/mesh/2011/MB_cgi?field=uid&term=D003937

[2] VINDICATE – Mnemonic for differential diagnosis (http://pgblazer.com/2010/05/vindicate-mnemonic-for-differential-diagnosis.html) at PG Blazer.com.

[3] Seccareccia, D. (Mar 2010). "Cancer-related hypercalcemia.". *Can Fam Physician* **56** (3): 244–6, e90-2. PMID 20228307. (http://www.ncbi.nlm.nih.gov/pmc/articles/PMC2837688/) (http://www.cfp.ca/content/56/3/244.full)

[4] (http://www.clinchem.org/cgi/reprint/34/12/2439.pdf) Lepage, R.; d'Amour, P.; Boucher, A.; Hamel, L.; Demontigny, C.; Labelle, F. (1988). "Clinical performance of a parathyrin immunoassay with dynamically determined reference values". *Clinical chemistry* **34** (12): 2439–2443. PMID 3058363.

[5] Bargren, A. E.; Repplinger, D.; Chen, H.; Sippel, R. S. (2011). "Can Biochemical Abnormalities Predict Symptomatology in Patients with Primary Hyperparathyroidism?". *Journal of the American College of Surgeons* **213** (3): 410–414. doi:10.1016/j.jamcollsurg.2011.06.401. PMID 21723154.

[6] Parathyroid Cancer Treatment (http://www.cancer.gov/cancertopics/pdq/treatment/parathyroid/HealthProfessional/page1) at National Cancer Institute. Last Modified: 03/11/2009

[7] Razzouk, D.; Mari, J. J.; Shirakawa, I.; Wainer, J.; Sigulem, D. (January 2006). "Decision support system for the diagnosis of schizophrenia disorders". *Brazilian Journal of Medical and Biological Research* **39** (1): 119–28. doi:/S0100-879X2006000100014. PMID 16400472.

[8] Hejlesen OK, Olesen KG, Dessau R, Beltoft I, Trangeled M (2005). "Decision support for diagnosis of lyme disease" (http://booksonline.iospress.nl/Extern/EnterMedLine.aspx?ISSN=0926-9630&Volume=116&SPage=205). *Studies in Health Technology and Informatics* **116**: 205–10. PMID 16160260. .

[9] "Evaluation of a Computer Assisted Decision Support System (DSS) for Diagnosis and Treatment of Ventilator Associated Pneumonia (VAP) in Intensive Care Unit (ICU)." (http://gateway.nlm.nih.gov/MeetingAbstracts/ma?f=102248792.html). *nih.gov.* . Retrieved 2008-10-03.

[10] "DiagnosisPro differential diagnosis reminder tool" (http://en.diagnosispro.com/). *diagnosispro.com.* . Retrieved 2008-10-03.

[11] http://www.visualdx.com

Further reading

* The *Merck Manual of Diagnosis and Therapy* has 11 index entries describing the topic as differential diagnosis.

Medical_diagnosis

Medical diagnosis (often simply termed **diagnosis**) refers both to the process of attempting to determine or identify a possible disease or disorder (and diagnosis in this sense can also be termed (medical) **diagnostic procedure**), and to the opinion reached by this process (also being termed (medical) **diagnostic opinion**). From the point of view of statistics the diagnostic procedure involves classification tests. It is a major component of, for example, the procedure of a doctor's visit.

The plural of diagnosis is *diagnoses*, the verb is *to diagnose*, and a person who diagnoses is called a *diagnostician*. The word *diagnosis* (English pronunciation: /daɪ.əɡˈnoʊsɪs/) is derived through Latin from the Greek word διαγιγνώσκειν, meaning to discern or distinguish.[1] This Greek word is formed from διά, meaning *apart*, and γιγνώσκειν, meaning *to perceive*.

Overview

Diagnostic procedure

A diagnosis, in the sense of diagnostic procedure, can be regarded as an attempt at classification of a an individual's condition into separate and distinct categories that allow medical decisions about treatment and prognosis to be made. Subsequently, a diagnostic opinion is often described in terms of a disease or other condition, but in the case of a wrong diagnosis, the individual's actual disease or condition is not the same as the individual's diagnosis.

A diagnostic procedure may be performed by various health care professionals such as a physician, physical therapist, chiropractor, healthcare scientist, dentist, podiatrist, nurse practitioner, or physician assistants. This article uses *diagnostician* as any of these person categories.

A diagnostic procedure (as well as the opinion reached thereby) does not necessarily involve elucidation of the etiology of the diseases or conditions of interest, that is, what *caused* the disease or condition. Such elucidation can be useful to optimize treatment, further specify the prognosis or prevent recurrence of the disease or condition in the future.

Diagnostic opinion

However, a diagnosis can take many forms.[2] It might be a matter of naming the disease, lesion, dysfunction of disability. It might be a management-naming or prognosis-naming exercise. It may indicate either degree of abnormality on a continuum or kind of abnormality in a classification. It's influenced by non-medical factors such as power, ethics and financial incentives for patient or doctor. It can be a brief summation or an extensive formulation, even taking the form of a story or metaphor. It might be a means of communication such as a computer code through which it triggers payment, prescription, notification, information or advice. It might be pathogenic or salutogenic. It's generally uncertain and provisional.

It should be noted that medical diagnosis in psychology or psychiatry is problematic. There are differing theoretical views toward mental conditions and few objective tests available for various major disorders (e.g., clinical depression), so a causal analysis with respect to symptomatology and disorder/disease is not always possible. As a result, most if not all mental conditions function as both symptoms and disorders. There are often functional descriptions provided for psychological disorders and these are vulnerable to circular reasoning due to the etiological fuzziness inherent of these diagnostic categories. (BDG, 2006)

Indication for diagnostic procedure

The initial task is to detect a medical indication to perform a diagnostic procedure. Indications include:

- Detection of any deviation from what is known to be normal, such as can be described in terms of, for example, anatomy (the structure of the human body), physiology (how the body works), pathology (what can go wrong with the anatomy and physiology), psychology (thought and behavior) and human homeostasis (regarding mechanisms to keep body systems in balance). Knowledge of what is normal and measuring of the patient's current condition against those norms can assist in determining the patient's particular departure from homeostasis and the degree of departure, which in turn can assist in quantifying the indication for further diagnostic processing.
- A complaint expressed by a patient.
- The fact that a patient has sought a diagnostician can itself be an indication to perform a diagnostic procedure. Therefore, in, for example, a doctor's visit, the physician may already start performing a diagnostic procedure by, for example, watching the gait of the patient from the waiting room to the doctor's office even before she or he has started to present any complaints.

Even during an already ongoing diagnostic procedure, there can be an indication to perform another, separate, diagnostic procedure for another, potentially concomitant, disease or condition. This may occur as a result of an incidental finding of a sign unrelated to the parameter of interest, such as can occur in comprehensive tests such as radiological studies like magnetic resonance imaging or blood test panels that also include blood tests that are not relevant for the ongoing diagnosis.

General components

General components, which are present in a diagnostic procedure in most of the various available methods include:

- Complementing the already given information with further data gathering, which may include questions of the medical history (potentially from other people close to the patient as well), physical examination and various diagnostic tests.
  A diagnostic test is any kind of medical test performed to aid in the diagnosis or detection of disease. Diagnostic tests can also be used to provide prognostic information on people with established disease.[3]
- Processing of the answers, findings or other results. Consultations with other providers and specialists in the field may be sought.

Specific methods

There are a number of methods or techniques that can be used in a diagnostic procedure, including performing a differential diagnosis or following medical algorithms.[4] In reality, a diagnostic procedure may involve components of multiple methods.[4]

Differential diagnosis

The method of differential diagnosis is based on finding as many candidate diseases or conditions as possible that can possibly cause the signs or symptoms, followed by a process of elimination or at least of rendering the entries more or less probable by further medical tests and other processing until, aiming to reach the point where only one candidate disease or condition remains as probable. The final result may also remain a list of possible conditions, ranked in order of probability or severity.

The resultant diagnostic opinion by this method can be regarded more or less as a diagnosis of exclusion. Even if it doesn't result in a single probable disease or condition, it can at least rule out any imminently life-threatening conditions.

Unless the provider is certain of the condition present, further medical tests, such as medical imaging, are performed or scheduled in part to confirm or disprove the diagnosis but also to document the patient's status and keep the patient's medical history up to date.

If unexpected findings are made during this process, the initial hypothesis may be ruled out and the provider must then consider other hypotheses.

Pattern recognition

In a pattern recognition method the provider uses experience to recognize a pattern of clinical characteristics.[4] It is mainly based on certain symptoms or signs being associated with certain diseases or conditions, not necessarily involving the more cognitive processing involved in a differential diagnosis.

This may be the primary method used in cases where diseases are "obvious", or the provider's experience may enable him or her to recognize the condition quickly. Theoretically, a certain pattern of signs or symptoms can be directly associated with a certain therapy, even without a definite decision regarding what is the actual disease, but such a compromise carries a substantial risk of missing a diagnosis which actually has a different therapy so it may be limited to cases where no diagnosis can be made.

Diagnostic criteria

The term *diagnostic criteria* designates the specific combination of signs, symptoms, and test results that the clinician uses to attempt to determine the correct diagnosis.

Some examples of diagnostic criteria are:

- Amsterdam criteria for hereditary nonpolyposis colorectal cancer
- McDonald criteria for multiple sclerosis
- ACR criteria for systemic lupus erythematosis

Clinical decision support system

Clinical decision support systems are interactive computer programs designed to assist health professionals with decision-making tasks. The clinician interacts with the software utilizing both the clinician's knowledge and the software to make a better analysis of the patients data than either human or software could make on their own. Typically the system makes suggestions for the clinician to look through and the clinician picks useful information and removes erroneous suggestions.[5]

Other diagnostic procedure methods

Other methods that can be used in performing a diagnostic procedure include:

- Usage of medical algorithms
- An "exhaustive method", in which every possible question is asked and all possible data is collected.[4]

Diagnostic opinion and its effects

Once a diagnostic opinion has been reached, the provider is able to propose a management plan, which will include treatment as well as plans for follow-up. From this point on, in addition to treating the patient's condition, the provider can educate the patient about the etiology, progression, prognosis, other outcomes, and possible treatments of her or his ailments, as well as providing advice for maintaining health.

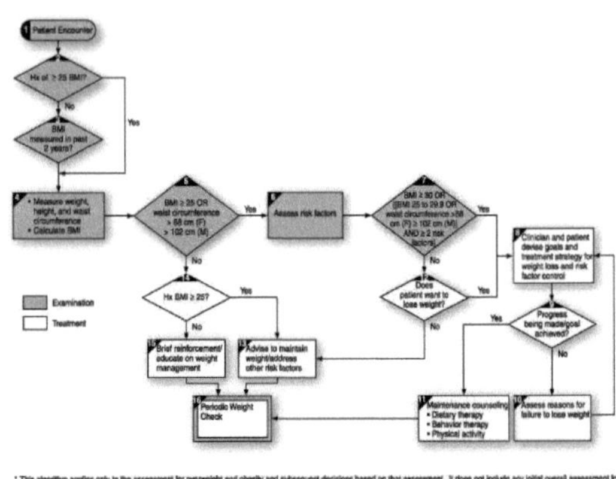

An example of a medical algorithm for assessment and treatment of overweight and obesity.

A treatment plan is proposed which may include therapy and follow-up consultations and tests to monitor the condition and the progress of the treatment, if needed, usually according to the medical guidelines provided by the medical field on the treatment of the particular illness.

Relevant information should be added to the medical record of the patient.

A failure to respond to treatments that would normally work may indicate a need for review of the diagnosis.

Additional types of diagnosis

Sub-types of diagnoses include:

Clinical diagnosis

> A diagnosis made on the basis of medical signs and patient-reported symptoms, rather than diagnostic tests

Laboratory diagnosis

> A diagnosis based significantly on laboratory reports or test results, rather than the physical examination of the patient. For instance, a proper diagnosis of infectious diseases usually requires both an examination of signs and symptoms, as well as laboratory characteristics of the pathogen involved.

Radiology diagnosis

> A diagnosis based primarily on the results from medical imaging studies. Greenstick fractures are common radiological diagnoses.

Principal diagnosis

> The single medical diagnosis that is most relevant to the patient's chief complaint or need for treatment. Many patients have additional diagnoses.

Admitting diagnosis

The diagnosis given as the reason why the patient was admitted to the hospital; it may differ from the actual problem or from the *discharge diagnoses*, which are the diagnoses recorded when the patient is discharged from the hospital.

Differential diagnosis

A process of identifying all of the possible diagnoses that could be connected to the signs, symptoms, and lab findings, and then ruling out diagnoses until a final determination can be made.

Diagnostic criteria

Designates the combination of signs, symptoms, and test results that the clinician uses to attempt to determine the correct diagnosis. They are standards, normally published by international committees, and they are designed to offer the best sensitivity and specificity possible, respect the presence of a condition, with the state-of-the-art technology.

Prenatal diagnosis

Diagnosis work done before birth

Diagnosis of exclusion

A medical condition whose presence cannot be established with complete confidence from either examination or testing. Diagnosis is therefore by elimination of all other reasonable possibilities.

Dual diagnosis

The diagnosis of two related, but separate, medical conditions or co-morbidities; the term almost always refers to a diagnosis of a serious mental illness and a substance addiction.

Self-diagnosis

The diagnosis or identification of a medical conditions in oneself. Self-diagnosis is very common and typically accurate for everyday conditions, such as headaches, menstrual cramps, and headlice.

Remote diagnosis

A type of telemedicine that diagnosis a patient without being physically in the same room as the patient.

Nursing diagnosis

Rather than focusing on biological processes, a nursing diagnosis identifies people's responses to situations in their lives, such as a readiness to change or a willingness to accept assistance.

Computer-aided diagnosis

Providing symptoms allows the computer to identify the problem and diagnose the user to the best of it's ability. Health screening begins by identifying the part of the body where your symptoms are located, the computer cross-references a database for the corresponding disease and presents a diagnosis. [6]

Overdiagnosis

The diagnosis of "disease" that will never cause symptoms, distress, or death during a patient's lifetime

Wastebasket diagnosis

A vague, or even completely fake, medical or psychiatric label given to the patient or to the medical records department for essentially non-medical reasons, such as to reassure the patient by providing an official-sounding label, to make the provider look effective, or to obtain approval for treatment. This term is also used as a derogatory label for disputed, poorly described, overused, or questionably classified diagnoses, such as pouchitis and senility, or to dismiss diagnoses that amount to overmedicalization, such as the labeling of normal responses to physical hunger as reactive hypoglycemia.

Retrospective diagnosis

The labeling of an illness in a historical figure or specific historical event using modern knowledge, methods and disease classifications.

Overdiagnosis

Overdiagnosis is the diagnosis of "disease" that will never cause symptoms or death during a patient's lifetime. It is a problem because it turns people into patients unnecessarily and because it can lead to economic waste (overutilization) and treatments that may cause harm. Overdiagnosis occurs when a disease is diagnosed correctly, but the diagnosis is irrelevant. A correct diagnosis may be irrelevant because treatment for the disease is not available, not needed, or not wanted.

Errors in diagnosis

Further information: Medical error

Causes and factors of error in diagnosis are:[7]

- the manifestation of disease are not sufficiently noticeable
- a disease is omitted from consideration
- too much significance is given to some aspect of the diagnosis
- the condition is a rare disease with symptoms suggestive of many other conditions
- the condition has a rare presentation

Lag time

When making a medical diagnosis, a *lag time* is a delay in time until a step towards diagnosis of a disease or condition is made. Types of lag times are mainly:

- *Onset-to-medical encounter lag time*, the time from onset of symptoms until visiting a health care provider[8]
- *Encounter-to-diagnosis lag time*, the time from first medical encounter to diagnosis[8]

History

The history of medical diagnosis began in earnest from the days of Imhotep in ancient Egypt and Hippocrates in ancient Greece. In Traditional Chinese Medicine, there are four diagnostic methods: inspection, auscultation-olfaction, interrogation, and palpation.[9] A Babylonian medical textbook, the *Diagnostic Handbook* written by Esagil-kin-apli (fl. 1069-1046 BC), introduced the use of empiricism, logic and rationality in the diagnosis of an illness or disease.[10] The book made use of logical rules in combining observed symptoms on the body of a patient with its diagnosis and prognosis.[11] Esagil-kin-apli described the symptoms for many varieties of epilepsy and related ailments along with their diagnosis and prognosis.[12]

The practice of diagnosis continues to be dominated by theories set down in the early 20th century.

See also

- Diagnosis codes
- Diagnosis-related group
- Diagnostic and Statistical Manual of Mental Disorders
- Doctor-patient relationship
- Etiology
- International Statistical Classification of Diseases and Related Health Problems (ICD)
- Medical classification
- Merck Manual of Diagnosis and Therapy
- Misdiagnosis and medical error
- Nosology
- Pathogenesis
- Pathology
- Preimplantation genetic diagnosis

Lists

- List of diseases
- List of disorders
- List of medical symptoms
- Category:Diseases

References

[1] "Online Etymology Dictionary" (http://www.etymonline.com/index.php?term=diagnosis). .

[2] Treasure, Wilfrid (2011). "Chapter 1: Diagnosis". *Diagnosis and Risk Management in Primary Care: words that count, numbers that speak.* Oxford: Radcliffe. ISBN 978-1846194771.

[3] Thompson, C. & Dowding, C. (2009) Essential Decision Making and Clinical Judgement for Nurses.

[4] Making a diagnosis, John P. Langlois, Chapter 10 in Fundamentals of clinical practice (2002). Mark B. Mengel, Warren Lee Holleman, Scott A. Fields. 2nd edition. p.198. ISBN 0-306-46692-9

[5] Decision support systems. 26 July 2005. 17 Feb. 2009 <http://www.openclinical.org/dss.html>

[6] WebMed Solutions. "Connection between onset of symptoms and diagnosis" (http://www.webmedicine.ca). . Retrieved 15 January 2012.

[7] Johnson, P. E.; Duran, A. S.; Hassebrock, F.; Moller, J.; Prietula, M.; Feltovich, P. J.; Swanson, D. B. (1981). "Expertise and Error in Diagnostic Reasoning". *Cognitive Science* **5** (3): 235–283. doi:10.1207/s15516709cog0503_3.

[8] Chan, K.; Felson, D.; Yood, R.; Walker, A. (1994). "The lag time between onset of symptoms and diagnosis of rheumatoid arthritis". *Arthritis and rheumatism* **37** (6): 814–820. PMID 8003053.

[9] Jingfeng, C. (2008). *Medicine in China.* pp. 1529–1534. doi:10.1007/978-1-4020-4425-0_8500.

[10] H. F. J. Horstmanshoff, Marten Stol, Cornelis Tilburg (2004), *Magic and Rationality in Ancient Near Eastern and Graeco-Roman Medicine,* p. 97-98, Brill Publishers, ISBN 90-04-13666-5.

[11] H. F. J. Horstmanshoff, Marten Stol, Cornelis Tilburg (2004), *Magic and Rationality in Ancient Near Eastern and Graeco-Roman Medicine,* p. 99, Brill Publishers, ISBN 90-04-13666-5.

[12] Marten Stol (1993), *Epilepsy in Babylonia,* p. 5, Brill Publishers, ISBN 90-72371-63-1.

External links

- The Merck Manuals Online Medical Library (http://www.merck.com/mmpe/)

Pericardium

Pericardium	
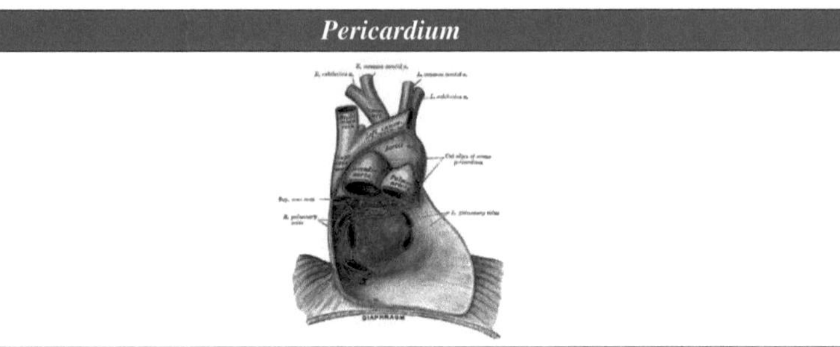 Posterior wall of the pericardial sac, showing the lines of reflection of the serous pericardium on the great vessels.	
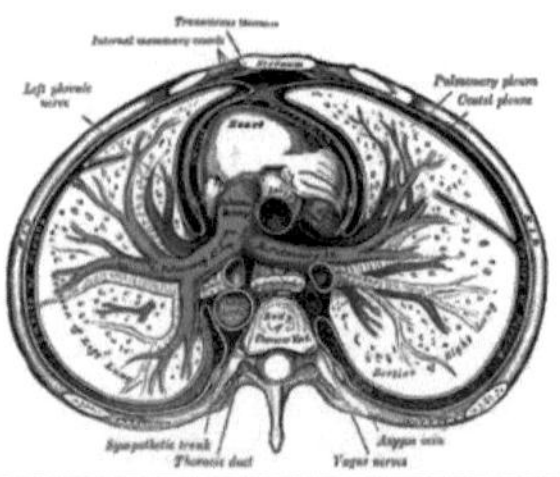 A transverse section of the thorax, showing the contents of the middle and the posterior mediastinum. The pleural and pericardial cavities are exaggerated since normally there is no space between parietal and visceral pleura and between pericardium and heart Paricardium is also known as cariac epidemis.	
Gray's	*subject #137 524* [1]
Artery	pericardiacophrenic artery
MeSH	*Pericardium* [2]

The **pericardium** (from the Greek περι, "around" and κάρδιον, "heart" /perikardion/) is a double-walled sac that contains the heart and the roots of the great vessels.

Layers

There are two layers to the pericardial sac: the outermost fibrous pericardium and the inner serous pericardium. The serous pericardium, in turn, is divided into two layers, the *parietal pericardium*, which is fused to and inseparable from the fibrous pericardium, and the *visceral pericardium*, which is part of the epicardium. The epicardium is the layer immediately outside of the heart muscle proper (the myocardium).

The visceral layer extends to the beginning of the great vessels, becoming one with the parietal layer of the serous pericardium. This happens at two areas; where the aorta and pulmonary trunk leave the heart and where the superior vena cava, inferior vena cava and pulmonary veins enter the heart.

In between the parietal and visceral pericardial layers there is a potential space called the pericardial cavity. It is normally lubricated by a film of pericardial fluid. Too much fluid in the cavity (such as in a pericardial effusion) can result in pericardial tamponade (compression of the heart within the pericardial sac). A pericardectomy is sometimes needed in these cases.

Functions

- Protection
- Lubrication

Anatomical relationships

- Surrounds heart and bases of pulmonary artery and aorta.
- Deep to sternum and anterior chest wall.
- The right phrenic nerve passes to the right of the pericardium.
- The left phrenic nerve passes over the pericardium of the left ventricle.
- Pericardial arteries supply blood to the dorsal portion of the pericardium.

Diseases/Abnormalities

- Pericarditis resulting in pericardial friction rub
- Pericardial effusion which may lead to cardiac tamponade.
- Cardiac Tamponade as a primary pathology following traumatic injury.

Relating topics

Pericardial sinus

Additional images

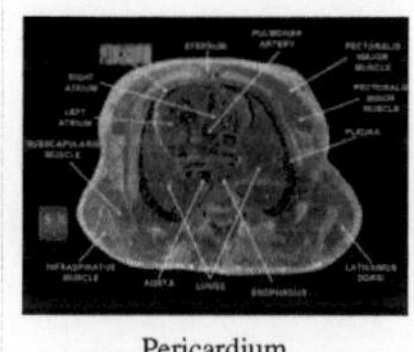

Pericardium

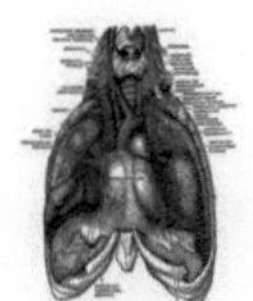

The phrenic nerve and its relations with the vagus nerve.

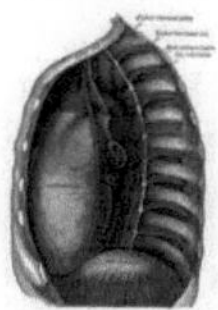

Thoracic portion of the sympathetic trunk.

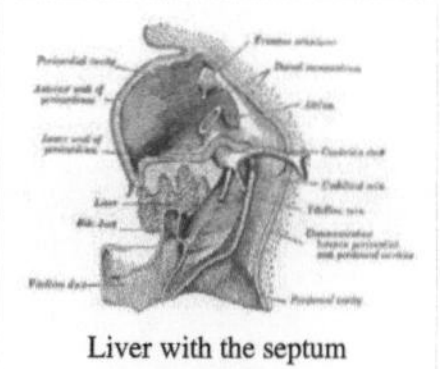

Liver with the septum transversum. Human embryo 3 mm. long.

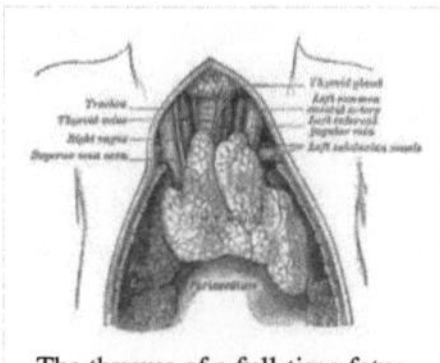

The thymus of a full-time fetus, exposed in situ.

External links

- SUNY Labs *21:st-1500* [3] - "Mediastinum: Pericardium (pericardial sac)"
- *thoraxlesson4* [4] at *The Anatomy Lesson* [5] by Wesley Norman (Georgetown University) (*heartpericardium* [6])

References

[1] http://education.yahoo.com/reference/gray/subjects/subject?id=137#p524

[2] http://www.nlm.nih.gov/cgi/mesh/2011/MB_cgi?mode=&term=Pericardium

[3] http://ect.downstate.edu/courseware/haonline/labs/l21/st1500.htm

[4] http://mywebpages.comcast.net/wnor/thoraxlesson4.htm

[5] http://home.comcast.net/~wnor/homepage.htm

[6] http://mywebpages.comcast.net/wnor/heartpericardium.jpg

Apex_of_the_heart

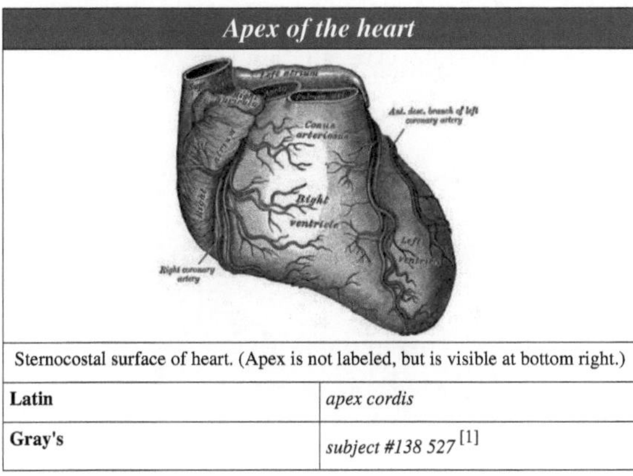

Sternocostal surface of heart. (Apex is not labeled, but is visible at bottom right.)	
Latin	*apex cordis*
Gray's	*subject #138 527* [1]

The **apex of the heart** is the lowest superficial part of the heart.

It is directed downward, forward, and to the left, and is overlapped by the left lung and pleura.

External anatomy

It lies behind the fifth left intercostal space, 8 to 9 cm from the mid-sternal line, slightly medial to the midclavicular line.

Alternately, it can be found about 4 cm below and 2 cm to the medial side of the left mammary papilla.

External links

- *Apex+of+heart* [2] at eMedicine Dictionary
- SUNY Labs *20:05-0104* [3] - "Heart: Sternocostal Surface of the Heart"
- Roche Lexicon - illustrated navigator, at Elsevier *02101.002-2* [4]

This article was originally based on an entry from a public domain edition of Gray's Anatomy. *As such, some of the information contained within it may be outdated.*

References

[1] http://education.yahoo.com/reference/gray/subjects/subject?id=138#p527

[2] http://www.emedicinehealth.com/script/main/srchcont_dict.asp?src=Apex+of+heart

[3] http://ect.downstate.edu/courseware/haonline/labs/l20/050104.htm

[4] http://www.tk-online.de/rochelexikon/pics/s02101.002-2.html

Auscultation

For the ancient monasterial worker, see Auscultare

<table>
<tr><td colspan="2" align="center">Auscultation</td></tr>
<tr><td colspan="2" align="center">Intervention</td></tr>
<tr><td colspan="2">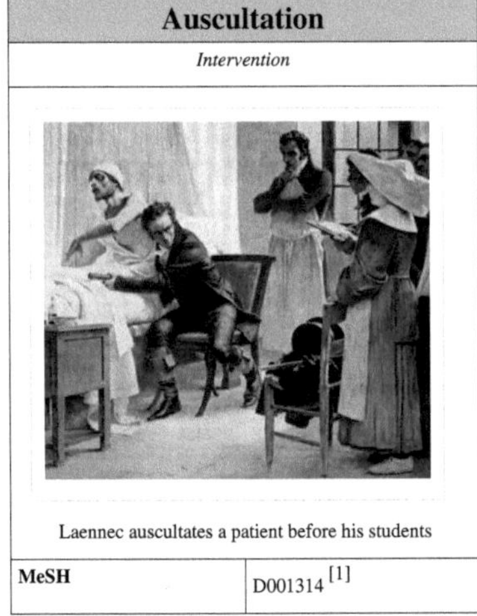</td></tr>
<tr><td colspan="2" align="center">Laennec auscultates a patient before his students</td></tr>
<tr><td>MeSH</td><td>D001314 [1]</td></tr>
</table>

Auscultation (based on the Latin verb *auscultare* "to listen") is the term for listening to the internal sounds of the body, usually using a stethoscope. Auscultation is performed for the purposes of examining the circulatory system and respiratory system (heart sounds and breath sounds), as well as the gastrointestinal system (bowel sounds).

The term was introduced by René-Théophile-Hyacinthe Laënnec. The act of listening to body sounds for diagnostic purposes has its origin further back in history, possibly as early as Ancient Egypt. Laënnec's contributions were refining the procedure, linking sounds with specific pathological changes in the chest, and inventing a suitable instrument (the stethoscope) in the process. Originally, there was a distinction between immediate auscultation (unaided) and mediate auscultation (using an instrument).

Auscultation is a skill that requires substantial clinical experience, a fine stethoscope and good listening skills. Doctors listen to three main organs and organ systems during auscultation: the heart, the lungs, and the gastrointestinal system. When auscultating the heart, doctors listen for abnormal sounds including heart murmurs, gallops, and other extra sounds coinciding with heartbeats. Heart rate is also noted. When listening to lungs, breath sounds such as wheezes, crepitations and crackles are identified. The gastrointestinal system is auscultated to note the presence of bowel sounds.

Electronic stethoscopes can be recording devices, and can provide noise reduction and signal enhancement. This is helpful for purposes of telemedicine (remote diagnosis) and teaching. This opened the field to computer-aided auscultation.

Auscultogram

The sounds of auscultation can be depicted using symbols to produce an auscultogram. It is used in cardiology training.[2]

See also

- Pericardial friction rub
- Heart sounds
- Breath sounds
- Triangle of auscultation
- Percussion (medicine)

References

[1] http://www.nlm.nih.gov/cgi/mesh/2011/MB_cgi?field=uid&term=D001314
[2] Constant, Jules (1999). *Bedside cardiology*. Hagerstwon, MD: Lippincott Williams & Wilkins. pp. 123. ISBN 0-7817-2168-7.

External links

- The Auscultation Assistant (http://www.med.ucla.edu/wilkes/intro.html), - "provides heart sounds, heart murmurs, and breath sounds in order to help medical students and others improve their physical diagnosis skills"
- MEDiscuss (http://www.mediscuss.org/content/respiratory-auscultation-tips-audio-mp3-examples-71.html) - Respiratory auscultation with audio examples
- Traditional Chinese medicine (http://www.365tcm.com/articles/diagnosing-methods-of-chinese-medicine.html) - Auscultation of Traditional Chinese medicine
- Blaufuss Multimedia (http://www.blaufuss.org) - Heart Sounds and Cardiac Arrhythmias
- http://www.andries.com - Commercial site, online auscultation training and a test instruction
- Thinklabs (http://www.thinklabsmedical.com) - Commercial site, digital stethoscopes
- Independent Stethoscope Review (http://www.forusdocs.com/reviews/Acoustic_Stethoscope_Review.htm) - Comparative review of stethoscopes, including frequency response graphs.

Article Sources and Contributors

Ph.eyes, Piano non troppo, Płyd, Rich Farmbrough, Rjwilmsi, Robodoc.at, SMcCandlish, Shawnc, Shd, Sqush101, Starwarp2k2, SteveW, Stwalkerster, Tagishsimon, The Epopt, Thetrista, Three-quarter-ten, Thumperward, Trgreer79, Trouble18, Tuggler, Una Smith, WhatamIdoing, Woohookitty, Wstclair, 132 anonymous edits

Medical_diagnosis *Source*: http://en.wikipedia.org/w/index.php?title=Medical_diagnosis *Contributors*: 4cecz4, Absolutezero273, Alex.tan, Allgoodnamesalreadytaken, Andrewpmk, Anonymaus, Arcadian, ArmadilloFromHell, Beland, BennyD, Betacommand, BigEars42, Bobblewik, BokicaK, Bongwarrior, Bozman007, Bushytails, Bwrs, COMPFUNK2, Cacycle, Canihaveacookie, Cervelo58, Cgingold, Charles Matthews, ChrisCork, CloudSurfer, Cnilep, Cremepuff222, Dacoutts, Davidruben, Deli nk, Demon 83, Discospinster, DoctorDW, DoctorDoctorGimmetheNews, Doczilla, Dr Wilf, Earthsound, Eclipse Anesthesia, Ed Poor, Eequor, El C, Erich gasboy, Erikpatt, EvelinaB, Excirial, F-402, Fences and windows, Fun2playlondon, Fuzbaby, Gavin.collins, Gfoley4, Gogo Dodo, Greetings, Earthling, Gveret Tered, Headlikeawhole, HendrixEesti, Hordaland, Hosim, Hugh2414, InfoCan, Iridescent, Irs550, J. Ash Bowie, JLaTondre, JPG-GR, Jagged 85, Jakeallenseo, Japanese Searobin, Jauerback, Jclemens, Jeff3000, Jesanj, Jfdwolff, Jlittlet, Jm34harvey, Jmh649, Johnkarp, Jon Awbrey, JonHarder, Jpmaytum, Juansempere, Kafziel, Kd4ttc, Keakealani, Klughammer, Kmadoc0, Kpjas, Kungming2, Kuru, Kwamikagami, Lawrancj, LeafPlacement, Lexor, Lightmouse, Lindsay658, LonelyMarble, Lumbercutter, Lynch1000s, MER-C, Mac, MacMog, Materialscientist, MattBan, MattKingston, Matthew Treder, Mendalus, Mercury, Metju, Mgiganteus1, Michael Hardy, Mikael Häggström, Mlawsky, Mlibby, Ncurrier, Nemu, Nescio, NickGorton, Nposs, Oddben, OldMonkeyPuzzle, Optimist on the run, Orenwhite, Osm agha, Osnimf, Paddles, Panthouse, Patriarch, Patrick, Pde, Petersam, Pgr94, PhnomPencil, Pinethicket, Pkubin, Plesiosaur, Polacrilex, Radomil, Raimundo Pastor, Ranveig, Rapidbi, Reginalafferty, Rg165309, Rich Farmbrough, Rjwilmsi, Rossami, SHCarter, Samgg, Sbi, ScottSteiner, SeyADiiDAyes, SiobhanHansa, Snoyes, Someone else, Stassats, SubDural12, Sundar, Supten, Taylornate, Template namespace initialisation script, The Thing That Should Not Be, Thingg, Three-quarter-ten, Ummuldrg, Una Smith, Versageek, Vincej, WhatamIdoing, Xndr, Xyz or die, Yosri, Zhenqinli, 142 anonymous edits

Pericardium *Source*: http://en.wikipedia.org/w/index.php?title=Pericardium *Contributors*: 28421u2232nfenfcenc, A little insignificant, Adville, Alan Liefting, Alex.tan, Anatomist90, Anim8cme, Arcadian, Aristolaos, Bemoeial, Carabinieri, Cburnett, Chanson101, Crohnie, Drminnesota, Ekko, ElBeeroMan, Emperorbma, EncycloPetey, Funny.pochi, Geni, Gwernol, Heidimo, JonHarder, Jonomacdrones, Joshuajohnlee, Kadellar, Katieh5584, Kdso, Kpjas, Ksheka, Lemonsky91, Lowellian, Mgiganteus1, Miniyazz, Nono64, Notheruser, Nyxie, Osm agha, PFHLai, Prissi, Quirk, RA0808, Renato Caniatti, Rmburkhead, Rohita, Sam Hocevar, ShabbatSam, Sheeana, Specter01010, Squirrels2nuts, Tahmmo, Tannim101, Template namespace initialisation script, Thescientist556, Unyoyega, Verkhovensky, Versus22, Vogon77, Wendell, Wouterstomp, 74 anonymous edits

Apex_of_the_heart *Source*: http://en.wikipedia.org/w/index.php?title=Apex_of_the_heart *Contributors*: Arcadian, Carl Daniels, D-rew, EncycloPetey, Goldom, GregorB, Kappa, Keilandreas, Kyleolm, Snalwibma, 13 anonymous edits

Auscultation *Source*: http://en.wikipedia.org/w/index.php?title=Auscultation *Contributors*: A. B., Alison.philp, AnjaManix, Arcadian, Brian0918, Centenarian, Dechetes, Dick Langer, Dimwight, Erich gasboy, Fandries, GregorB, HendrixEesti, High Contrast, Izvora, Jack-A-Roe, Jason Quinn, Jimjamns, Jmh649, KrakatoaKatie, LadyofShalott, Madhero88, Maneroof, Mild Bill Hiccup, MrOllie, NeilN, Nephron, Patrick, Pch123, Ph.eyes, Pkubin, Pol098, Power.corrupts, Rich Farmbrough, Rishigupta02445, Sharkface217, Sole Soul, Thys.cronje, Tjajkovskij, Una Smith, Wakablogger2, Wasbeer, 35 anonymous edits

Image Sources, Licenses and Contributors

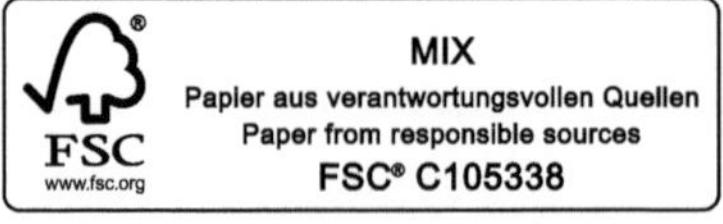

Printed by Books on Demand GmbH, Norderstedt / Germany